I0134967

The Superpowers of Superfoods:

Eat Your Way to Better Health Using the Natural Power of Foods

ERRYN O'CAIN, PharmD.

© Copyright 2021 Publishers Dailey, LLC.
All rights reserved.
The content contained within this book may not be reproduced, duplicated or transmitted without direct written permission from the author or the publisher.

Under no circumstances will any blame or legal responsibility be held against the publisher, or author, for any damages, reparation, or monetary loss due to the information contained within this book, either directly or indirectly.

Legal Notice:

This book is copyright protected. It is only for personal use. You cannot amend, distribute, sell, use, quote or paraphrase any part, or the content within this book, without the consent of the author or publisher.

Disclaimer Notice:

Please note the information contained within this document is for educational and entertainment purposes only. All effort has been executed to present accurate, up to date, reliable, complete information. No warranties of any kind are declared or implied. Readers acknowledge that the author is not engaged in the rendering of legal, financial, medical or professional advice. The content within this book has been derived from various sources. Please consult a licensed professional before attempting any techniques outlined in this book.

By reading this document, the reader agrees that under no circumstances is the author responsible for any losses, direct or indirect, that are incurred as a result of the use of the information contained within this document, including, but not limited to, errors, omissions, or inaccuracies.

DEDICATION

To Christon, Darin and Leah, my three reasons for everything.

CONTENTS

ACKNOWLEDGMENT

To my beloved people from that pharmacy in Chickasaw. Thank you for entrusting your lives to me. Taking part in your healthcare journeys for over a decade has taught me valuable lessons that I will forever carry with me.

INTRODUCTION

Do you find it difficult to break free from your unhealthy eating habits? Or does nighttime snacking, emotional eating, skipping breakfast, or junk-food binges sound like a normal trend for you? Well, whether your answer is a "Yes" or "No," the truth is that we all do practice some of these bad eating habits despite knowing fully well that they are extremely bad for our health. But even science agrees that it is not totally our fault.

Here is how it works. Basically, our taste buds are genetically wired to desire high-calorie and high-fat foods. In all honesty, most highly processed foods are produced to taste a lot better than nature. Perhaps, this explains why we are most likely to choose a juicy hamburger over lettuce!

Resisting such temptations takes great willpower! A study conducted in 2010 discovered that when rats were regularly given fast food to eat, their brain chemistry began to transform negatively. These rats became obese and had no control over how they ate. They would eat fatty foods even when they were not hungry. When they were transferred and placed on a healthy diet, these rats actually refused to eat. This study, just like the countless research, proved that food could be just as addictive as drugs.

Unfortunately, these foods only end up causing us to develop health problems or simply increase our risk of developing suboptimal health conditions like lethargy, obesity, chronic pain, and other bodily ailments. They weaken our immune system and make us more vulnerable to chronic diseases like cancer, diabetes, and coronary diseases.

Now we have clearly stated just how much winning this fight over unhealthy foods is a total necessity for us to live healthier and disease-free lives. But still, our dream of eating healthy seems somewhat impossible since we live in a world where highly processed foods and junk foods are constantly and readily available.

Luckily for us, there is hope and good news, as the addiction goes both ways! In the same way, unhealthy fast foods can be addictive as hard drugs; you can also get addicted to nature's superfoods when you start eating them more. Let's assume you hate mushrooms presently. The more you eat them regularly, the more you'll begin to enjoy them.

Of course, this isn't as simple as it sounds, especially when you don't even know the game rules. That's exactly why this book was written to be your ultimate guide on this journey to developing better, more healthy eating habits!

This book's contents cover the various foods we consider to be "superfoods," as well as how specifically each of them will affect and benefit your body. This valuable knowledge will also help you know and understand the exact weapons (superfoods) you need to succeed and achieve the best results in this journey. But you know we cannot fight and win without knowing exactly how to use our weapons, right? Hence, the book also provides you essential information about incorporating these healthy food items into your diet. I have compiled some quick, easy, and highly effective superfood recipes that can make the process easier for you.

As a pharmacist who has acquired over a decade of experience working with people to help treat diseases, manage their health, and improve their health outcomes, I am extremely passionate about assisting people in reducing the number of medications they take and understanding that many diseases are reversible and preventable through proper diet and exercise. There is an array of natural foods power-packed with essential nutrients designed to keep our bodies healthy and functioning properly. This book goes into great details about the many health benefits of these so-called "superfoods" and provides tips and recipes to incorporate these natural medicines into our daily diets. Let's first find out what superfoods are!

1

WHAT'S SO SUPER ABOUT SUPERFOODS?

Undoubtedly, you're most likely familiar with the term "superfoods" as it is an overused word in the market and media today. Now, you would agree that for something to have earned such a label, then surely it must be an exceptional thing, isn't it? Let's focus on exploring what "superfoods" are and what makes them so super?

Interestingly, there is no official or exact definition of what "superfoods" are. Thus, we tend to examine them from the perspective of their benefits.

Superfoods are often considered to be nutrient powerhouses produced by Mother Nature. This simply implies that these foods have been specially singled out as being power-packed with important nutrients that enhance a healthy eating pattern. In most cases, superfoods are usually plant-based, from berries and veggies to fruits and seeds. Some fish and dairy also count.

Apparently, the powers that these superfoods offer emerge from a force deep within them. They house large quantities of essential nutrients that the body needs.

Essentially the point we are trying to make here is that these superfoods are accredited with the "super" title because they are loaded with nutrients that play a great role in promoting good health, improving immunity, and preventing disease. These nutrient-dense foods do not only make you feel and look great, but they also help in reducing your risk of certain chronic health conditions. Superfoods are also well known for effectively protecting the body organs from toxins. They also help lower cholesterol and regulate your body's metabolism. All of the super benefits we just stated are simple generalizations so let's be more specific!

Superfoods contain antioxidants, healthy fats, fiber, and vitamins and minerals. Each of these nutrients is essential in its own way. Hence to prove just how super superfoods are, we will critically analyze some of these nutrients individually.

Vitamins and Minerals

Let's start with vitamins and minerals. Vitamins and minerals perform hundreds of roles in the body.

To keep itself active and alive, the human body performs different important activities like producing rich red blood to carry nutrients and oxygen, churning out chemical messengers that deliver instructions from one organ to another, and much more. However, for it to perform these functions effectively, your body requires at least 30 vitamins, minerals, and other dietary components that it cannot manufacture on its own in sufficient amounts. And like you might have guessed by now, the high vitamin and mineral content present in superfoods can help your body perform these functions more effectively.

Beyond this, vitamins and minerals convert food into energy and increase the body's energy levels. They also strengthen and boost up your immune system, thereby warding off diseases and keeping you healthier.

These nutrients also help you shore up your bones, repair any cellular damage and heal wounds due to the combinations of calcium, vitamin D, vitamin K, magnesium, and phosphorus contained in some superfoods.

With vitamins and minerals present in superfoods, they have the power to promote heart health and even reduce the effects of aging. Vitamins help promote a healthy and beautiful skin complexion and improve your nails and hair health. So, imagine enhancing both your outer and inner body health all in one go; how great is that?

Also, these two nutrients, especially minerals (folic acid), help prevent congenital disabilities. Thus, as a woman, the consumption of effective superfoods early in your pregnancy helps prevent brain and congenital spinal disabilities in your child.

Vitamins and minerals are often called micronutrients because your body needs only tiny amounts of them. What's very interesting about this is that failing to get even those small quantities virtually means you are automatically increasing your risk of developing certain diseases.

Antioxidants

Antioxidants are natural molecules that are available in many superfoods. Their major function is to help neutralize the free radicals in our body system. These free radicals are the natural byproducts of energy production that can cause serious problems in our bodies. The antioxidant molecules decrease or reverse the negative effects of free radicals, especially those closely associated with health problems like coronary diseases, cancer, arthritis, stroke, emphysema, and Parkinson's disease. The molecules improve your immunity and can prevent such conditions from developing.

In the same way, antioxidants help prevent and repair the inevitable occurrence of oxidative stress in the body. This process mostly damages cells and causes aging. Antioxidants also help in decreasing inflammation. There are many more benefits that antioxidants deliver, but we will explore those as we progress further in this book.

Healthy Fats

You might be thinking, "but how can fats be healthy?" Indeed, they are, and eating the right amount and kind of fat like those present in most superfoods won't necessarily make you fat. The type of fat that is not beneficial to your body in any way is Trans fats, an artificial kind of fat mainly found in partially hydrogenated oils. Trans fats are another reason to avoid processed food.

The type of fat that makes superfoods "super" are available in two main forms: unsaturated and saturated fat. Unsaturated fats are oils that are liquid at room temperature. So, you can envision it to be something like olive oil. On the other hand, saturated fats are solid at room temperature, such as a stick of butter or glob of coconut oil. We need both kinds in our diet, but most should come from unsaturated fats. You see, for those vitamins and antioxidants we discussed earlier, you need fats to help you absorb some of them, especially the fat-soluble vitamins like vitamin A, D, E, and K.

Also, some superfoods offer a type of unsaturated fat called Omega-3 fats which is important for our optimum nerve, brain, and heart function. It even helps to reduce your risk of heart disease.

Phytochemicals

It was earlier mentioned that most superfoods are plant-based. This automatically means that they contain phytochemicals which are the chemical compounds that occur naturally in plants. They are usually produced to protect plants against different environmental threats, including pollution, predatory insects, and diseases.

Now phytochemicals were previously known as the non-essential nutrients found in plant-based foods, and by non-essential, they are not of any usefulness to human life. However, a growing body of studies and research has provided evidence that suggests phytochemicals are actually beneficial to your health in numerous ways.

To start with, phytochemicals can protect us from cancer and cardiovascular diseases. To do this, the phytochemical contents inhibit cell proliferation and angiogenesis, which simply mean the growth of new blood vessels. These two terms are trademarks of cancer. In the case of people who have already been diagnosed with cancer, the phytochemicals block carcinogens while inducing programmed cell death in cancer cells and protecting your cells against DNA damage. A special type of phytochemical, Saponins also interferes with cell replication, including cancer cells.

Apart from protection against cancer, phytochemicals regulate nitric oxide, help in relaxing blood vessels, and increase blood flow. It also helps in reducing symptoms of menopause.

Fiber

Fiber is another rich nutrient that makes many superfoods "super." Most of us probably have heard that fiber aids digestion and helps to prevent or relieve constipation. That is very true, but how exactly does this nutrient achieve that?

The presence of fiber in these superfoods helps increase your stool's weight and size and then softens it. As such, it becomes easier to pass out, decreasing your chance of constipation. If the reverse is the case and you have loose, watery stools, the fiber content may solidify the stool by absorbing the water and adding bulk to the stool. It's the perfect "drug" to help keep you regulated!

The fiber contents in superfoods offer many other health benefits like helping you to easily maintain a healthy weight and reducing your risk of diabetes, heart disease, and some types of cancer, such as colorectal cancer.

Of course, just like every other nutrient we've previously discussed, there is a thin but very important line between getting enough of this nutrient and getting too much to harm you in different ways like promoting intestinal gas, abdominal bloating, cramping, etc.

Luckily by consuming most superfoods, we cannot exceed the right amount we need. Nevertheless, many of us deny our body the right amount of fiber it requires to function normally by consuming more refined or processed foods like pulp-free juices, pasta, canned fruits and vegetables, non-whole-grain cereals, etc. Unlike superfoods, the processed food is lower in fiber. During the refining process, the outer coat (bran) of these grains, fruits, and others is removed, lowering the fiber content. See why you totally need to switch and take advantage of the super benefits of superfoods?

You will see these 6 nutrients and even more as we analyze some specific superfoods that are quite effective. However, just before we dive deeply into the overview and health benefits of the various superfoods discussed in this book, you must understand that no single superfood can offer us all the nutrition, health benefits, and energy we need to nourish ourselves. Simply put, superfoods are not cure-all foods.

2

LEMON AND LIMES

Suppose we should ask anyone, including you reading this, about the two fruits from the citrus family that can be said to be interchangeable. No doubt your answer will definitely include lemons and limes! Although these two fruits have different appearances and flavors, nutritionally, they both share very similar profiles and potential health benefits.

Both lemons and limes have a long history of use in traditional medicine. They each contain antioxidants, vitamins, and minerals and provide a range of health benefits we will soon be analyzing.

Nutritional Breakdown of Lemons and Limes

We already stated that lemons and limes share similar nutritional profiles. Now you will see detail in the following table. Please note that these nutrients reflected here are present in a whole lemon or lime and not in the juice.

Nutrient	Lemon	Lime
Calorie	24.4	20.1
Carbs (Total)	7.83g	7.06 g
Fiber	2.35 grams	1.88 grams
Sugars	2.1 g	1.13 g
Vitamin B9 (Folate)	9.24 mcg	5.36 mcg
Calcium	21.8 mg	22.1 mg
Potassium	116 mg	68.3 mg
Vitamin C	44.5 mg	19.5 mg

From this table, you can confirm that lemon and lime contain similar content of nutrients, though with some slight variations in their quantities. Lemons are a richer source of vitamin C and folate than limes, but more vitamin A is present. To some extent, lemons have fewer carbohydrates and more protein compared to limes.

Health Benefits of Lemons and Limes

Different parts of lemons and limes can offer great medicinal benefits to your health when consumed in the right amounts.

Aids in Weight Loss

As superfoods, lemons, and limes are often known as great weight loss foods, and there are many reasons for this. They contain a special kind of antioxidant, Polyphenols. This antioxidant molecule is said to hold off weight and body fat gain.

A scientific study was conducted on mice placed on fattening diets and were fed with polyphenols extracted from the peel of lime and lemon. They gained less weight and body fat than other mice who were not placed on this diet with time. Maybe that is enough proof, but we can't really be sure since the study was just conducted on animals. No scientific research has proven that lemon, or lime, can cause weight loss in humans.

Nevertheless, some scientists believe that these superfoods change how your body processes the fat and improves its insulin response.

This, in turn, improves your insulin resistance. Lemons and limes also offer your body's required hydration and oxygen while even stabilizing its pH levels to make you feel lighter, have more energy, and be healthier overall.

Prevents and Treats Urinary Tract Infections

We most likely might have heard before of lemons and limes being promoted for weight loss but do you know that using these superfoods in meals or juice can help prevent and cure urinary tract infections (UTI)? Well, UTIs usually develop due to bacterial infections. Thus, the condition is typically treated with prescribed antibiotics.

Similarly, natural superfoods like lemons and limes are often as powerful and effective as antibiotics. With their richness in vitamin C and antioxidants, these two substances act as diuretic agents, encouraging your urinary bladder to expel more urine frequently and thus, increasing the chances of the bacterial toxins being flushed out of the body.

To prevent urinary tract infections naturally, lemons and limes can also cause the pH of your blood and urinary tract to change from acidic to alkaline, causing unfavorable conditions for these opportunistic bacteria to grow.

Lowers Your Cholesterol Level

Finding a way to incorporate lemons and limes into the foods you eat can lower your cholesterol and improve the armada of fats floating through your bloodstream. These superfoods are rich in pectin, a type of soluble fiber that lowers Low-Density Lipoprotein (LDL). The LDL is the harmful cholesterol-carrying particle that contributes to artery-clogging atherosclerosis, which in simpler terms means the hardening of the arteries. This condition can eventually cause heart disease, heart attacks, and strokes.

Lemons and limes can help decrease these risks when used as a natural remedy against high cholesterol. According to experts, lemon and lime seem to work best when used along with garlic or honey.

Helps Treat Dandruff

Dandruff is not an illness of any sort, but it can certainly be very annoying and frustrating to deal with. What exactly causes dandruff?

In most cases, dandruff is usually caused by the presence of Malassezia, which is a yeast-like fungus that feeds on the oils available on your scalp. When this fungus becomes excessive, they cause your scalp to dry out and become irritated. Apart from this, dandruff can also be caused by the hair products you use. Now, how do lemon and lime come in to save the day?

The superfoods offer vitamin C, citric acid, flavonoid, and iron, all of which are essential to hair and scalp health. Since citric acid is a natural pH adjuster for the scalp, it can eliminate the scalp's excess oils that build up and cause flakes. Vitamin C and other powerful antioxidants in these citrus fruits also help strengthen hair follicles and promote collagen production to help repair the damaged skin cells in your scalp.

If you check the ingredients used in the most effective shampoos, you will discover that they include either lemon or lime or both. The use of these fruits also contributes to the shampoos' fragrant smell.

Helps Prevent Peptic Ulcers

Peptic ulcers are open sores that develop on your stomach's inside lining and the upper portion of your small intestine (Mayo clinic, 2020, para.1). Instead of taking acid-reducing medications, using superfoods like lemon and lime that are quite rich in ascorbic acid can be a better option for preventing peptic ulcers. Although the juice from these two fruits is very acidic, it can help neutralize the acid in your stomach when mixed in small amounts with water. Having such an alkalizing effect actually helps protect the stomach from peptic ulcers. Furthermore, if you deal with acid-reflux or indigestion, drinking a glass of warm water with two teaspoons of lime juice about 30 minutes before meals may help prevent these gastric symptoms.

Promotes Healthy Gums and Fresh Breath

Swollen, bleeding gums can be treated using lemon and limes in the right amount or manner. You will notice that much antiseptic mouthwash has lemon-based ingredients in them. This is because the antimicrobial effects of this fruit can kill the microbes causing the infection and resulting swelling. Basically, these fruits act as mouth fresheners but with more effective benefits. They also tend to stimulate saliva, which helps to prevent dry mouth.

Prevents Kidney Stones

There is no way we'll talk about kidney stones without including Limes and lemons. Wonder why?

Well, firstly, you should understand that kidney stones are small lumps that form when waste products build up in your kidneys. This condition is quite common, and those who experience them once usually tend to develop it repeatedly. But the presence of citric acid and vitamin C in these two superfoods can increase your urine volume and urine pH. This will, in turn, help break up or prevent the formation of specific types of kidney stones.

Offers Anti-Aging Skin Benefits

In the previous chapter, we discussed just how much superfoods containing vitamins could be great for skin care. Well, lemons and lime contain the right amounts of vitamin C that can help prevent your skin from wrinkling and promote collagen production to make your skin springy and full. Lemon and lime juice can also be placed on the skin as a peel to lighten dark spots, freckles, and other forms of hyperpigmentation. Waking up each morning to a warm glass of water with lemons will deliver that youthful glow we all desire!

How to Include Lemons and Limes in Your Meal

Not only are lemons and limes great superfoods with effective health benefits, but they also have a unique, pleasant taste and smell that can take your foods and drinks to the next level when you use them!

Of course, it is well known that lemons and limes are rarely eaten raw, but they are used to flavor many sweet and savory dishes. So, here are a few tips on how you can use them in your meals:

1. Extract the lemon or lime juice and make a refreshing lemonade or lime beverage by adding water and sugar to the fresh juice. You can try freezing them about 24 hours before to make the extraction even easier. A little precaution; make sure you drink any lemon or lime beverage with a straw because it helps prevent the acid in the juice from touching your teeth and eroding tooth enamel.

2. You can squeeze the lemon or lime juice into your soup, sauces, or even pasta to boost their taste. Add the juice only at the end of the cooking time or after the dish has been cooked to minimize vitamin C loss.

3. Add lemon juice to your steamed vegetables to help them keep their bright colors and enhance their flavor.

4. You can cut down on the amount of salt used on your food by adding lemon or lime instead to enhance the food's flavor. Both the zest and juice can make fancy finishing salts!

5. You can add lemon or lime juice to the cooking water to make your rice fluffier.

6. Use lemon or lime as a garnish, in the form of a slice, cheek or wedge served with your meals and drinks.

7. Lemon and lime juice can also be used as a marinade to tenderize meat.

8. Use lemon or lime juice in place of vinegar while making simple salad dressings. You can combine it with olive oil, salt, pepper, and any other flavoring agents you like.

9. Do you know you can make buttermilk with lemon and lime juice? Just add fresh lemon juice to your regular milk and let it start to look a little curdled. You can also add them to yogurt.

10. You can use both the juice and zest of lemons and limes in

baked goods and desserts like cake or doughnuts to provide them with light, fresh flavors.

11. Thanks to their high vitamin C content, you can also use lemon or lime juice to prevent discoloring the flesh of already-cut fruits and vegetables that oxidize quickly when exposed, like avocados and even lemons themselves.

12. You can make lemon or lime oil from the zest of the lemon or lime. They taste fantastic when used in salad dressing.

Now that you have all the adequate information about these superfoods, it's time to shop for lemons and limes! Make sure that they are bright yellow and green, respectively. They should also have a shine on their skin.

3

BELL PEPPERS AND CHILIS

Bell peppers and chilis are siblings of the capsicum annuum species from the same nightshade family. However, these superfoods are opposites. So, while bell peppers are typically known as big sweet peppers that come in a rainbow of colors, chilis are notable for their hot flavors.

Apart from being sweet and flavorful, we also know that bell peppers have zero-heat, which is why they can be eaten raw and fresh and will still give you that satisfying crunch and taste. They can also be stuffed and cook with other ingredients to build flavor and substance into many different dishes.

At the opposite end, chili peppers are primarily used as a spice. But exactly what causes this spicy flavor? Well, Capsaicin, which is the main bioactive plant compound in chili peppers, is responsible for their unique, pungent taste! (Arnarson, 2019, para. 4). Chilis can be cooked or dried and powdered.

Though chili pepper mostly comes in red and sometimes green when they are unripe, bell peppers are found in an array of bright colors, including green, yellow, orange or red, brown, white, or even purple in rare cases. In terms of flavor, it varies with color. Actually, every bell pepper starts green, but color changes and their sweetness increases depending on how long they're allowed to ripen on the vine. Basically, the colors and flavors of bell peppers are determined by the variety of the pepper plant and ripeness stage when picked. (Mike, 2020, para. 2)

Obviously, there is a great difference between bell peppers and chili peppers regarding their colors, flavor, and size. Nevertheless, they share similar nutrients that offer exceptional health benefits that you most likely never thought of before!

Generally, these two superfoods are low in calories and exceptionally rich in vitamins A, B, and C and other antioxidants, making them an excellent addition to a healthy diet. There is so much more, so keep reading!

Nutritional Breakdown of Bell Peppers and Chilis

These low-calorie superfoods are made of mostly water. Though the nutrients vary in quantity, each consists of carbs with a small portion of fat and protein.

The nutrients in 3.5 ounces (100 grams) of raw bell peppers and chili pepper measure as follows:

Nutrient	Bell Peppers	Chili Peppers
Calories	31	6
Water	92%.	88%
Protein	1 gram	0.3 grams
Carbs	6 grams	1.3 grams
Sugar	4.2 grams	0.8 grams
Fiber	2.1 grams	0.2 grams

Fats	0.3 grams	0.1 grams

Health Benefits of Bell Peppers and Chilis

Powers up your Immune System

Thanks to their high content of vitamins, specifically Vitamins A and C, bell peppers and chilis have been greatly valued as powerful immunity boosters. Vitamin A is essential for supporting your body's primary defense areas such as your respiratory passages, urinary tract, and intestinal tract. By increasing the strength of these systems, your body easily finds ways to avoid becoming ill. Vitamin C also helps form and maintain connective and cardiovascular tissues, ensuring that your body remains strong.

Improves Heart Health

In the previous chapter, we already established that people with high levels of oxidized LDL are more likely to develop heart disease because the LDL type of cholesterol is prone to adhering to arteries' walls when it is oxidized. That tendency can result in the condition known as atherosclerosis, and eventually heart disease. Demonstrating their power as a superfood, bell peppers contain high levels of quercetin and zeaxanthin, two antioxidants that can help fight low-density oxidation lipoprotein (LDL). This ensures the blocking of any tendency that can lead to the development of any heart disease.

Chili peppers also contain riboflavin and niacin, responsible for maintaining healthy cholesterol levels, which automatically reduces heart disease risk. Studies have shown that chili peppers can also protect fats in your blood against free radicals (Rikesh, para. 20)

Both chili and bell peppers contain a great amount of potassium and folate, which, when combined effectively, support your cardiovascular system. and reduce your chances of developing heart disease. Potassium is also an important mineral. It helps relax your blood vessels, enabling blood to flow more easily through your body.

Promotes a Reduced Risk of Cancer

A considerable amount of research shows the value of bell peppers, especially the red ones, for fighting certain cancers (Bray, 2019, para.1). This is because this superfood contains cancer-fighting nutrients like vitamin C, E, and lycopene. With these anti-cancer agents packed within them, bell peppers are especially effective against prostate, breast, and lung cancers. Some scientists and researchers have reduced the size of different cancer tumors by taking advantage of the unique combination of nutrients packed in red bell peppers.

The same thing is applicable with chili peppers. According to the American Association for Cancer Research, the capsaicin and antioxidants present in chili peppers can kill cancer cells in leukemia and prostate cancer. For example, in prostate cancer, capsaicin reduces prostate cancer cells' growth by triggering a depletion of cancer cell lines' primary types.

Helps Fight Cold and Flu

The presence of capsaicin in chilis gives them the therapeutic antibacterial properties to fight chronic sinus infections, chest colds, coughs, excess mucus, and bronchitis.

So, here is how the magic happens! Chili pepper encourages coughing, which forces the mucus to get moving and eventually out, thereby clearing nasal and throat pathways and removing germs and irritants out of your body.

Headaches are also a common symptom of the flu and colds. The capsaicin in chili pepper can also help prevent the trigeminal nerve pain and decrease the calcitonin gene-related peptide (CGRP), both of which are responsible for creating headache pain. (Rinkesh, para. 5)

Improves Eye Health

Two carotenoid enzymes, Lutein, and zeaxanthin are found in relatively high amounts in bell peppers. A good number of studies have proven that the consistent consumption of foods rich in such carotenoids improves your eye health. The natural antioxidants protect your retina, which is the light-sensitive inner wall of your eye, from oxidative damage. These enzymes lower your risk of developing both cataracts and macular degeneration, which are the most common visual impairments caused by aging and infection. All in all, incorporating bell peppers into your diet may help lower your risk of visual impairments.

Helps in Treating Anemia

Red blood cells are vital in our body as they, among other things, help to carry oxygen from the lungs to other parts of the body. But what happens when there are no red blood cells to perform this essential task?

Anemia! This is a health condition that occurs when the number of red blood cells circulating in the body decreases (Lam, 2020, para. 1). In fact, it is the most common blood disorder. Chili peppers are a natural remedy that can be used to treat this condition often caused by iron- and vitamin deficiency.

Since chili peppers are rich in iron and copper, they help new cell formation. Chili peppers also contain folic acid and vitamin B supplements, both keys for treating anemia symptoms and producing healthy red blood cells.

Fights Inflammation

By now, you can conclude that Capsaicin is a medicated "superhero" in chili peppers. This time, we will focus on its valuable characteristics of being a potent anti-inflammatory agent. Basically, it inhibits substance P, a neuropeptide responsible for inflammatory processes that cause irritation, swelling, pain, etc. For this reason, capsaicin is believed to be a potential treatment for several sensory nerve disorders, such as arthritis pain, diabetic neuropathy, and psoriasis.

To support this claim, a study was conducted where animals treated with a substance that caused inflammatory arthritis responded well to a diet high in capsaicin. Due to this diet, the animals experienced a delayed development of arthritis and a significant inflammation decrease throughout their bodies. You will see capsaicin used as the active ingredient in over-the-counter analgesic ointments and pain patches.

How to Include Bell Peppers and Chilis in Your Meals

There are plenty of ways to cook these beautiful superfoods. But before we get into that, remember, don't cook them on high heat for a prolonged time because that will make them lose all their nutritional goodness!

Bell Peppers
1. Bell peppers are perfect for serving alongside dips, like a sour cream dip or spicy cream cheese dip.
2. Bake them by stuffing them up with delicious fillings.
3. You can dice and top them on home-made pizzas before baking or add them to an omelet before you fold it.
4. Add the pepper into your pasta sauce, soups, or chicken and salad.
5. Cut the bell peppers into chunks and use them to make veggie kebabs.
6. Brush the bell peppers with olive oil and sprinkle on a little salt, then grill them.
7. Toss bell pepper into the wok the next time you are cooking a stir-fried meal.
8. You can also try stacking slices of bell pepper into your wraps and sandwiches.

Chili peppers
1. You often see chili peppers roasted or grilled whole, or halved. They can also be dried or crushed for blending with other foods. Now here is how you can include them in your meals.
2. You can make a hot sauce, and there are many ways to cook

up a hot sauce!

3. Chop and add chili to your pasta.
4. When dried and grounded, you can add the chili pepper to chutneys.
5. Create a chili jam that goes well with a slice of delicious cheese!
6. Use chili pepper to complete the ingredients in your uncooked or cooked salsa to make your taste buds explode!
7. Use them to make chili poppers by filling them with cheese or other ingredients if you like.

Looking for a natural way to deal with some of your health issues? As you can see, bell peppers and chilis are an easy, tasty incorporation into any meal. Enjoying the sweet flavor or having a slight burn on your tongue or a teary eye might be worth its amazing health benefits!

4

ORANGES, WATERMELONS AND BLUEBERRIES

Oranges, watermelons, and blueberries are undoubtedly three of the most popular fruits around the world today. If you want to promote a healthy start for your day, these fruits are integral parts of an ideal healthy breakfast that you should eat. But don't take our word for it just yet! You will soon see for yourself just how much of an all-star nutritional superfood each of these fruits is.

Let's start with oranges! Now, just like lemons and limes that we discussed before; oranges belong to the citrus family. However, they are most popular because of their natural sweetness and the diversity in their uses and types (Megan Ware, 2019, para.2). Oftentimes, when we think of oranges, the first benefit that springs through our minds is that they are an excellent source of vitamin C! Indeed, they are terrific sources of this nutrient, but you might be surprised to find out that they offer much more health benefits than this. Not to worry, you will get to know about them soon. But just so you know, a typical orange should have smoothly textured skin and be firm and heavy for its size. These are usually the oranges with higher juice content than those that are either spongy or lighter in weight (ETIMES, 2019, para. 2)

Now, if you're in search of the most effective superfood to help you stay hydrated, especially during summer, watermelons are definitely a great option to consider. True to their name, watermelons contain around 90% water. They also contain other essential nutrients like vitamins, minerals, and antioxidants, all of which offer very effective health and medicinal benefits. But you know it is not just about their high level of nutrients. Watermelons contain natural sugars, which makes them super delicious.

Lastly, we have Blueberries! Blueberries are kings of antioxidant superfoods (Leech, 2019, para. 14). Sounds like an exaggeration? Well, that's an argument for later. Let's first find out where these tiny nutritional powerhouses come from. The blueberry bush is the flower-like shrub that produces these berries, giving them their blue-ish, purple hue. Surprisingly, these fruits usually first appear in green, then as they ripen deepen to purple and blue. Blueberries are packed with impressive health benefits and are the most nutrient-dense of all berries. It is highly recommended that everyone has a serving of at least 1/2 cup of blueberries every day.

Nutritional Breakdown of Oranges, Watermelons, and Blueberries

From the overview you just read, you will notice that each of these superfoods is low in calories and high in nutrients. Here is the breakdown.

One medium-sized orange has:

Calories	60	Carbs	15.4 grams
Fiber	3 grams	Calcium	6% of your daily recommended amount of Calcium
Sugar	12 grams	Potassium	237 milligrams
Water	85%		
Vitamin A	14 micrograms		
Vitamin C	70 milligrams		

A 1 cup serving of diced watermelon has the following nutrients.

Calories	46	Water content	139 g
Total fat	0.23 grams	Calcium	11 milligrams (1.1 % DV)
Carbohydrates	11.48 g	Iron	0.36 mg (2 % DV)
Dietary fiber	0.6 g (2.4 percent DV)	Vitamin C	12.3 mg (20.5 % DV)
Protein	0.93 g (1.86 percent DV)	Vitamin A	865 international units (IU) (17.3 % DV)
Sugars	9.42 g	Magnesium	15 mg (3.75 % DV)

Nutrient	Blueberries
Calories	84
Fat	0.5g
Carbohydrates	21g
Sodium	1.5mg
Fiber	3.6g
Sugars	15g
Protein	1g
Vitamin C	14.4mg

Health Benefits of Oranges, Watermelons, and Blueberries

Before we get started, you must understand that each of these three fruits has the potential of offering you the following benefits in their unique own ways.

Lowers Cholesterol

The antioxidants in blueberries, with the largest part being, anthocyanins are strongly linked to reduced levels of oxidized LDL (low-density lipoprotein) or "bad" cholesterol. These nutrients have been proven to be very helpful when it comes to preventing oxidative damage to "bad" LDL cholesterol. In the previous chapters, we have discussed how the oxidation of "bad" LDL cholesterol can cause different heart diseases.

Similarly, Phytosterols, which are one of the plant compounds in watermelons, can also help manage low-density lipoprotein (LDL) or "bad" cholesterol. A study carried out by US and Canadian researchers also revealed that a class of compounds found in oranges and other citrus peels called Polymethoxylated Flavones (PMFs) have the potential to lower cholesterol more effectively than some prescription drugs, and without side effects.

Regulates Blood Pressure

High blood pressure is another risk factor that can cause heart diseases. With the help of Vitamin B6 and magnesium packed in them, Oranges help support the production of hemoglobin and, at the same time, keep your blood pressure under check. Watermelon also contains citrulline, an amino acid that may increase nitric oxide levels in the body. This nitric oxide helps your blood vessels expand, which lowers blood pressure. This antioxidant, along with lycopene, may also help reduce the stiffness and thickness of artery walls common in obese and postmenopausal women. In a 2012 study, researchers found that watermelon extract reduced blood pressure in and around the ankles of middle-aged people with obesity and early hypertension (Ware, 2019, para. 9).

Like you might have guessed already, the superhero blueberries antioxidant can also help prevent high blood pressure.

Helps Prevent Cardiovascular Diseases

Due to anthocyanin content, blueberries may help prevent hard endpoints like heart attacks and other chronic cardiovascular diseases. A study in 93,600 nurses discovered that those with the highest intake of anthocyanins — the main antioxidants in blueberries — were at a 32% lower risk of heart attacks than those with the lowest intake.

Promotes Skin Health and Prevent Hair Damage

This is not the first time we mention improved skin and hair health. Like most superfoods, we will be exploring in this book, Oranges, Watermelons, and Blueberries are rich in Vitamin C and A, which are essential for your skin and hair. The body needs Vitamin C to produce collagen, a protein that keeps your hair strong and your skin supple and good-looking.

Beyond this, the antioxidant effects of these fruits can protect your skin from free radical damage, usually due to aging. Vitamin A also promotes wound healing and helps to create and repair your damaged cells. Vitamin C and A are the best skin- and hair-care products that can keep you looking young.

Controls your Blood Sugar

Oranges, Watermelons, and Blueberries provide moderate amounts of sugar compared to other fruits. However, the fiber content in these fruits help by keeping blood sugar levels under control. Its natural fruit sugar, fructose, can help keep blood sugar levels from rising too high after eating oranges. Its glycemic index is 40, which is considered to be low in sugar.

Similarly, the bioactive compounds in blueberries tend to outweigh the sugar's negative impact on blood sugar control. Research also suggests that anthocyanins in blueberries can help improve insulin sensitivity and glucose metabolism, which will in turn help to lower your body system's risk of metabolic syndrome and type 2 diabetes.

Now, this does not mean you can eat excessive amounts of oranges, watermelons. Eating too much can very well cause a spike insulin and may even lead to an increase in your body weight.

Offers Anti-inflammatory Benefits

By now, we understand that inflammation is a key driver of many chronic diseases like rheumatoid arthritis. These three fruits are rich in inflammatory-fighting antioxidants like Vitamin C, lycopene, Cucurbitacin E, and anthocyanins, which may help lower inflammation and oxidative damage, especially for those with rheumatoid arthritis.

Now for a less chronic condition like muscle soreness and fatigue, which is driven partly by local inflammation and oxidative stress in your muscle tissue, the amino acid, Citrulline, as well as Blueberry supplements, can help in minimizing muscle soreness and tightness. So, if you are an athlete or just a normal fitness enthusiast, you should consider incorporating these three superfoods into your diets to protect your muscles and joints.

Decreases Risk of Different Types of Cancers

Oranges, Watermelons, and blueberries are all excellent sources of

Vitamin C which is a powerful antioxidant that helps to get rid of free radicals, the unstable molecules that cause damage to our DNA. Oranges specifically contain D-limonene, a compound that helps prevent cancers like lung cancer, skin cancer, and even breast cancer.

Another plant compound, lycopene, present in watermelons, is also associated with a lower risk of some types of cancer, but the study results are mixed. While some studies linked lycopene intake with a lower risk of cancers of the digestive system, some other studies have linked the compound with a lower risk of prostate cancer.

Essentially, the lycopene compound reduces cancer risk by lowering the insulin-like growth factor (IGF), a protein involved in cell division. High IGF levels are linked to cancer (Jennings, 2018, para. 8).

As for blueberries; they are believed to have one of the highest antioxidant levels. As such, they can neutralize some of the free radicals that tend to damage your DNA.

Promotes a Healthy Brain

Oxidative stress doesn't just affect your heart. It can also accelerate your brain's aging process, thereby negatively affecting brain function. However, consuming any or all of these three fruits in the right quantity tends to benefit aging brain neurons, leading to cell signaling improvements. So, for instance, it may help delay the onset and progression of Alzheimer's disease.

Generally, these three fruits can help maintain your brain function and improve memory. Their antioxidant content also helps the areas of your brain that are essential for intelligence.

Helps you Stay Hydrated

Drinking water is an important way to keep your body hydrated. As we can confirm from the nutritional breakdown, these fruits, most especially watermelon, have a high-water content and can help keep you hydrated.

How to Include these Superfoods in Your Meals

Oranges

1. Oranges are a healthy snack that you can eat up quickly to give yourself that unique mid-day boost. Just make sure to eat the orange once you cut it up. This is because Vitamin C gets destroyed fast when exposed to air.

2. Make fresh orange juice! To extract more juice, try squeezing the oranges when they are at room temperature. The fresh orange juice usually lasts for 2-3 days if kept in a clean, tightly sealed bottle or jar.

3. You can also wash and freeze a whole orange in the freezer, then shred it with a grater once frozen (no need to peel it). Sprinkle the shredded orange on top of your salad, ice cream, soup, smoothies, noodles, pasta sauce, rice, sushi, fish dishes, etc.

4. Use the orange peels to make an herbal tea. It can actually help with stomach cramps and also act as an appetite stimulant.

5. You can use fresh orange juice to make syrup for your pancakes. Just simmer equal parts of it with water and sugar until the mixture becomes thick.

Watermelons

1. Just like oranges, you can eat up your watermelon fruits once you cut. Nevertheless, here are some diverse ways to incorporate watermelons into your meals and drinks.

2. Make a refreshing drink or cocktail from your watermelons.

3. Do you know you can grill your watermelon? Just cut it into wedges, brush them with olive oil and sprinkle with salt and pepper. Afterward, place it on your hot grill for about 90sec per side. Then serve it with crushed chili and a drizzle of lime juice and honey.

4. Use your watermelons to make mouth-watering salsa. Simply chop the watermelon into pieces and mix it with onions, bell

and jalapeno peppers, lime juice, and a sprinkle of salt and pepper. Then eat your newly-made salsa with tortilla chips.

5. Use either fresh or frozen watermelon to make smoothies. Simply cut your watermelon into cubes, and blend with your favorite fruits. You can try adding strawberry, Greek yogurt, fresh ginger, and honey to the combination. Then blend them well, pour and enjoy!

6. Use your watermelon as a "no-bake" cake and cover it with lite whipped cream.

Blueberries

1. Simply squeeze the juice from the berries and then drink the juice straight!

2. Make super sticky but not icky Blueberry Jam. You can always use them on your toasts. Tastes yummy!

3. Fill your ice cube tray with smaller blueberries or even blueberry juice and stick them in the freezer until they are fully frozen.

4. You can also add blueberries to your favorite smoothie recipe.

5. You can enjoy blueberries in your pancakes by simply adding a handful of them into your pancake batter. Then cook your pancakes all the way through.

6. To make blueberry muffins, add a handful of blueberries to your muffin batter and mix thoroughly. Fill your already greased muffin tins with the blueberries-filled batter and bake.

7. Use blueberries to make pies and then freeze them uncooked!

5

SUNFLOWER AND PUMPKIN SEEDS

Have you ever heard of the phrase, "Small but mighty"? Well, Sunflower and Pumpkin seeds are the perfect examples to describe that phrase in all of its fullness. Though they may come as tiny, tasty seeds, these superfoods are powerhouses of lots of valuable nutrients. Before we get deep into that, let's start with a quick overview of both groups of seeds.

Technically, sunflower seeds are the fruits of the sunflower plant (Helianthus annuus). They are usually harvested from the plant's large flower heads. You can harvest up to 2,000 seeds from a single sunflower head. Quite a lot, isn't it? Now about their taste; Sunflower seeds tend to have a mild, nutty flavor which is usually accompanied by a firm but tender texture.

Pumpkin seeds, on the other hand, are flat, oval-shaped green seeds that are usually picked from the flesh of a pumpkin. They are quite a common ingredient in Mexican cuisine.

Snacking straight off the sunflower or pumpkin seeds or roasting them to enhance their flavor is becoming quite a popular delicacy today. However, many of us may not realize that these tiny seeds are packed with important nutrients and offer many impressive health benefits beyond their sweet taste! So just how real are these claims? Let's find out!

Nutritional Breakdown of Sunflower and Pumpkin Seeds

The main nutrients in 1 ounce (30 grams or 1/4 cup) of shelled, dry-roasted sunflower seeds are as follows:

Calories	163	Niacin	10% of the RDI
Total Fat	14 grams	Pantothenic acid	20% of the RDI
Protein	5.5 grams	Magnesium	9% of the RDI
Carbs	6.5 grams	Iron	6% of the RDI
Fiber	3 grams	Zinc	10% of the RDI
Vitamin E	37% of the RDI	Copper	26% of the RDI
Vitamin B6	11% of the RDI	Manganese	30% of the RDI
Folate	17% of the RDI	Selenium	32% of the RDI

One ounce (28 grams) of shell-free pumpkin seeds contains:

Calories	151	Manganese	42% of the RDI
Fiber	1.7 grams	Magnesium	37% of the RDI
Carbs	5 grams	Iron	23% of the RDI
Protein	7 grams	Zinc	14% of the RDI
Fat	13 grams (6 of which are omega-6s)	Copper	19% of the RDI
Vitamin K	18% of the RDI	Phosphorus	33% of the RDI

Note that Pumpkin seeds have more proteins than peanuts.

Health Benefits of Sunflower Seeds

Strengthens Your Immune System

To maintain a good healthy lifestyle, having a strong immune system is a necessity. Thanks to the vitamin E, zinc, and selenium in them, sunflower and pumpkin seeds are great immune boosters. Now, let's break them down!

Vitamin E serves as a powerful antioxidant that enhances immune responses to prevent free radicals from damaging healthy cells in your body. Zinc helps the body to maintain and develop immune cells. Lastly, Selenium plays a vital role in reducing inflammation and boosting overall immunity.

So, imagine having those three powerful elements combined into one! There is no doubt that these seeds should be included in your well-balanced diet.

Improves Your Heart Health

Sunflower seeds are especially rich in unsaturated fatty acids. These fats are what we can refer to as "heart-friendly" fats. Now, the fatty acids and magnesium in the sunflower seeds block an enzyme that causes your blood vessels to constrict, thus enabling these vessels to relax and eventually lowering your blood pressure level.

This implies that you also get the added benefit of lowering your risks of developing cardiovascular diseases, high cholesterol, and high blood pressure by a regular consumption of sunflower seeds.

Helps in Maintaining a Healthy Weight

Sunflower seeds are packed with plenty of fiber and protein, which are essential nutrients for reducing pounds and/or maintaining a healthy weight. How exactly do they achieve this?

Both nutrients help make us feel full for a longer time, thereby forcing us to reduce our food intake and finally reducing the number of calories we tend to consume normally.

The fiber content also promotes good digestion, which is another great factor to check off when maintaining a healthy weight.

Boosts Your Energy Levels

Sunflower seeds are powerhouses of energy. They are rich in Vitamin B1 (Thiamine), which helps break down carbohydrates, proteins, and fats present in our food into instant energy that keeps us very active.

The presence of Selenium also increases blood flow and delivers more oxygen to your body. These two functions also help to keep us energized throughout the day.

Reduces Sugar Levels

Consuming Sunflower seeds is a great way to keep your blood sugar levels in control, especially if you are dealing with type 2 Diabetes Mellitus. The plant compound chlorogenic acid in the seeds is partially responsible for this blood-sugar-lowering effect. So if you are a diabetes patient, you can add Sunflower seeds to spice up your healthy diet!

Since these two superfoods share certain common nutrients, there are bound to be similarities in health benefits delivered by the two groups of seeds, as we can see from the nutritional breakdown. Take, for instance, improving your heart health, and lowering blood sugar levels. Nevertheless, pumpkin seeds are associated with specific but very important health benefits that we cannot help but put great emphasis on! Now that we've gotten that out of the way let's find out what these unique benefits are.

Health Benefits of Pumpkin Seeds

Reduces Inflammation in Arthritis

Pumpkin seeds are natural sources of antioxidants like carotenoids and vitamin E. These antioxidants can help protect your cells from harmful free radicals. This, in turn, reduces inflammation, especially in people with arthritis. In one study, pumpkin seed oil reduced inflammation in rats with arthritis without giving them any side effects. However, when you give the same set of animals the anti-inflammatory drug, they experience adverse effects. Can you see another piece of evidence that proves that you should sometimes try to pick superfoods like pumpkin seeds over-medicated drugs?

Reduces Risks of Cancers

Due to their high antioxidant activity and high lignan content, pumpkin seeds may help reduce risks of certain types of cancers such as colon, breast, lung, and stomach cancers. A German study on postmenopausal women revealed that eating pumpkin seeds reduces breast cancer risk (Dhanorkar, 2020, para.3). Further test-tube studies also found that a supplement containing pumpkin seeds had the potential to slow down the growth of prostate cancer cells (Jane Brown, 2018, para. 4)

Promotes Sleep and Prevents Insomnia

Have trouble sleeping at night? You might want to consider taking some pumpkin seeds with a small number of carbohydrates like a piece of fruit. Quite surprising, isn't it?

Well, Pumpkin seeds are a rich source of tryptophan, an amino acid that can help promote sleep (Jane Brown, 2018, para.10). It has been used to treat chronic insomnia. When the body gets the right amount of tryptophan, it converts the amino acid into serotonin, the "feel-good" or "relaxing" hormone, and melatonin, the "sleep hormone." So, in simpler terms; Tryptophan aids the body in the production of melatonin, the hormone that causes you to sleep.

Just in case you still can't believe this claim, here is a shred of evidence - a study published in 2005 in Nutritional Neuroscience suggested that consuming tryptophan from a gourd seed alongside a carbohydrate source was comparable to pharmaceutical grade tryptophan for the treatment of insomnia (Olsen, 2018 para.15). A seed as powerful as drugs but with no side effects; what can be more super?

Helps Relieve Symptoms of Benign Prostatic Hyperplasia

Benign prostatic hyperplasia (BPH) is when the prostate gland enlarges, causing urination problems. Research has proven that taking pumpkin seeds or their products as supplements can be a safe and effective treatment for BPH symptoms such as redness, itching, and pain in the prostate gland area.

One theory reveals that dihydrotestosterone, a powerful metabolite of testosterone, builds up in the prostate and causes it to grow. Thus, the phytochemicals in pumpkin seeds may block prostate growth by reducing dihydrotestosterone's effects on the prostate glands. They may also block testosterone's conversion into dihydrotestosterone (McDermott, 2016, para. 4). Also, you should keep in mind that Pumpkin seeds are an age-old cure for irritated or overactive bladder conditions.

Improve Sperm Quality

Having low zinc levels as a man causes an increased risk of reduced sperm quality and infertility. However, consuming the right amount of pumpkin seeds which are a rich source of zinc, may help solve this problem and further improve your sperm quality. Some studies suggest that they may also protect human sperm from damage caused by chemotherapy and autoimmune diseases.

Apart from their high zinc content, pumpkin seeds are also high in antioxidants that can contribute to healthy testosterone levels also leading to improved overall fertility levels and reproductive function, especially in men.

How to Include these Superfoods in Your Meals

Now that you have been exposed to the surprisingly great benefits packed in these seemingly small seeds, it's time to experience and enjoy them. Fortunately for us, we can easily incorporate these seeds into our meal.

1. First of all, sunflower and pumpkin seeds can be eaten either raw or roasted, salted, or unsalted.
2. To roast them properly, first, boil the seeds in salt water and wipe them. Then drizzle them with oil and salt and roast them in an oven at 320F for 10 minutes.
3. You can add them to smoothies, Greek yogurt, and fruit.
4. Sprinkle them into soups or cereals and top your salads with sunflower or pumpkin seeds.
5. You can also use any of the two seeds as an ingredient when baking sweet or savory loaves of bread and cakes.
6. Make homemade granola with either pumpkin or sunflower seeds, a mixture of nuts, and some dried fruits.

7. Brush the seeds with olive oil, season with cumin and garlic powder, and bake until brown and toasted.
8. Just like peanut butter, you can make your pumpkin or sunflower seed butter by blending the seeds whole and raw in a food processor until smooth.

6

MUSHROOM, ONIONS, AND BROCCOLI

As you know, vegetables are packed with essential nutrients. But certain vegetables are blessed with a range of extraordinary health benefits for humans. Mushrooms, onions, and broccoli belong to that set of superfoods.

Many don't realize that mushrooms, including crimini mushrooms, are actually a kind of fungus. Did somebody just say, "but Fungi aren't supposed to be eaten?" Well, maybe yes, but mushrooms are edible fungi that are quite popular for their delicate flavor and meaty texture. Now note that though there are around 2,000 edible varieties of mushrooms available today, there are also many varieties of poisonous mushrooms that are quite hard to distinguish from the edible ones. For this reason, it is not recommended to source mushrooms from the wild. Rather you should always buy from a reliable grocery store or market. The most common types you will find in grocery stores are shiitake, portobello, crimini, button or white mushroom, oyster, enoki, beech, maitake. You may not be aware, but almost every ancient civilization has used mushrooms for thousands of years because of their healing properties. The Ancient Egyptians even called the superfood "the plant of immortality." (Oberst, 2016). And perhaps they are right to say so because mushrooms are a rich, low-calorie source of fiber, protein, and antioxidants that can provide several important nutrients.

Green vegetables are not left off this list! Broccoli is undoubtedly one of the foremost foods that are said to be packed with the most nutritional punch of any vegetable. Not only is it a nutritional powerhouse full of vitamins, minerals, fiber, and antioxidants, but broccoli is also well known for being a hearty and tasty vegetable. This edible green plant belongs to the cruciferous family, making it relatives with cauliflower, cabbage, and kale.

Another vegetable that can help you stay away from medicated drugs and doctor's appointments is Onions. Like mushrooms, onions' medicinal properties have been recognized to be very effective for treating different ailments since ancient times. Onions belong to the Allium family of plants, which also includes chives, garlic, and leeks. Now, we all know onions vary in size, shape, color, and flavor. In terms of color, the most common types are usually red, yellow, and white. However, the taste of these vegetables tends to differ depending on how people grow and consume them. So, they range from sweet and juicy to sharp, spicy, and pungent. Due to the common knowledge that chopping onions causes watery eyes, most people tend to think that they improve our eyes' health. Well, maybe those assumptions are right, but you may never know unless you stick with us as we uncover some potential science-backed health benefits of this superfood! But first, let's see just how much nutrients each of these superfoods contain.

Nutritional Breakdown of Mushroom, Onions, and Broccoli

Though there are many varieties of mushrooms, most offer about the same quantities of the same nutrients per serving, regardless of their shape or size. The table below shows each nutrient-packed in a 96-g cup of whole, raw mushrooms.

Calories	21.1	Sodium	4.8 mg
Protein	3.0 g	Zinc	0.5 mg
Carbs	3.1 g	Copper	305 mcg
Calcium	2.9 mg	Selenium	8.9 mcg
Iron	0.5 mg	Vitamin C	2.0 mg
Magnesium	8.6 mg	Vitamin D	0.2 mg
Phosphorus	82.6 mg	Folate	16.3 mcg
Potassium	305 mg	Choline	16.6 mg

See how much nutrient is loaded in one cup (91 grams) of raw broccoli:

Carbs	6 grams	Vitamin K	116% of the RDI
Protein	2.6 gram	Vitamin B9 (Folate)	14% of the RDI
Fat	0.3 grams	Potassium	8% of the RDI
Fiber	2.4 grams	Phosphorus	6% of the RDI
Vitamin C	135% of the RDI	Selenium	3% of the RDI
Vitamin A	11% of the RDI		

Typical raw onions are very low in calories, with tiny amounts of protein and fat packed in them. The main nutrients in 3.5 ounces (100 grams) of raw onions are:

Calories	40
Water	89%
Protein	1.1 grams
Carbs	9.3 grams
Sugar	4.2 grams
Fiber	1.7 grams
Fat	0.1 grams

Health Benefits of Mushrooms, Onions, and Broccoli

Lowers risk of cardiovascular disease.

Mushrooms are rich in fiber, potassium, and vitamin C, all of which decrease your risk of heart diseases. Potassium content can help moderate your blood pressure by lessening your blood vessels' tension, decreasing hypertension risk. The American Heart Association (AHA) recommends reducing salt intake in the diet and eating more potassium-rich foods. This is because potassium helps in reducing the negative impact that sodium can have on your body. Beta-glucans, a type of fiber that occurs in the cell walls of many types of mushrooms, have also been proven to be effective for lowering blood cholesterol levels to a certain extent.

Broccoli also improves your heart health in its own variety of ways, with a major focus on reducing elevated "bad" LDL cholesterol and triglyceride levels, which are the major risk factors for heart disease. Like mushrooms, broccoli is also packed with soluble fiber, which binds with bile acids in the digestive tract, making excreting cholesterol out of the body easy. According to a research exercise by the Institute of Food Research, a particular variety of broccoli can help reduce the blood LDL-cholesterol levels by 6 percent (TNN, 2020, para. 3)

Onions have also been linked to improving cardiovascular health. A 2019 review found that quercetin, a compound in onion skin, had the power to lower blood pressure when the researchers extracted it and administered it as a supplement. Still, the study did not examine the potential effects on blood pressure if the onions are eaten as part of the diet rather than quercetin in supplement form (Ware, 2018, para.).

Prevents Different Types of Cancers

Mushrooms, onions, and broccoli are also very beneficial because of their apparent cancer-fighting powers. Mushrooms specifically contain a class of proteins called lectins, which have the ability to bind to abnormal cells and cancer cells and then label them for destruction by our immune system. Some scientists have done a lot of research about the links between eating mushrooms and breast cancer prevention. In one study of 2,000 women conducted by researchers from the University of Western Australia in Perth, women who consumed at least a third of an ounce of fresh mushrooms every day were discovered to be 64% less likely to develop breast cancer. That's more than average!

Researchers have also examined allium vegetables like onions extensively in relation to cancer, especially stomach and colorectal cancers. Though they have found out that a diet with higher onion consumption has been linked to a decreased risk of colorectal cancers than a diet with low onion consumption, experts do not fully understand the exact mechanism by which some compounds in onions can prevent cancer. Nevertheless, some studies have linked these cancer-fighting properties to the sulfur compounds and flavonoid antioxidants present in onions. For example, onions provide Allium, a sulfur-containing compound that has been shown to decrease tumor development and slow the spread of ovarian and lung cancer in test-tube studies. Onions also contain fisetin and quercetin, both of which may inhibit tumor growth (Kubala, 2018, para. 5).

Some studies also revealed that broccoli might also have anti-cancer properties suitable for reducing prostate, breast, and uterine cancer risk. One of its major key components, a phytochemical known as sulforaphane, is said to be effective in lowering these types of cancer (Shubrook, 2019, para. 6).

Helps in Managing Diabetes

Mushrooms, onions, and broccoli are excellent choices of food if you have diabetes. Mushrooms and broccoli are quite rich in dietary fiber. Beta-glucan, a form of soluble dietary fiber in mushrooms, helps your body regulate blood sugar, reducing the risk of type 2 diabetes. For those who already have it, the fiber may help reduce blood glucose levels. Oyster and shiitake mushrooms are believed to have the most effective beta-glucans. Now for eating broccoli, one study showed reduced insulin resistance in persons with type 2 diabetes who eat broccoli sprouts daily for 1 month. The Dietary Guidelines for Americans recommend that adults consume 22.4–33.6 g of dietary fiber each day, depending on sex and age. Consuming mushrooms and broccoli can certainly contribute an impressive amount to a person's daily requirement of fiber.

Apart from fiber, specific compounds, such as quercetin and sulfur compounds in onions, have also been found to possess antidiabetic effects. The compounds, most especially quercetin, have been shown to interact with cells in the small intestine, pancreas, skeletal muscle, fat tissue, and liver to control blood sugar regulation in the whole body.

Helps to Achieve Weight Loss

Mushrooms and broccoli are also great for weight loss because of their rich fiber content. With these dietary fibers in them, these superfoods help curb overeating, increase satiety, and reduce appetite. In one study, researchers gave people less meat and more mushrooms in place of meat. After just one year, people reported feeling healthier, and they lost a lot of weight. As stated earlier, you can also try replacing the amount of meat you consume with mushrooms and broccoli.

Treat Headaches and Mouth Sores

Drinking onion juice can help you get rid of the symptoms of sore throats. The sulfur compounds contained in this superfood help fight mucus overload and promote its expulsion from your airways. This benefit isn't just limited to treating sore throat. Onions are also powerful natural antibiotics that can fight off both viral and bacterial infections, thereby curing common cold-related illnesses like cough, high fever, and headaches. It can also boost your body's immunity such that it becomes less susceptible to these infections.

Decreases Risk of Developing Alzheimer's

Mushrooms contain various special antioxidants that may inhibit the buildup of amyloid-beta and tau in the brain. Those two foreign-looking words are basically proteins that are hallmarks of Alzheimer's disease. A study by researchers in Singapore who used data on 663 Chinese men and women over 60 found out that the older men and women who ate mushrooms several times a week were at reduced risk of developing mild cognitive impairment (Bakalar, 2019, para.4). This means that to a certain extent, eating mushrooms may reduce the risk for mild cognitive impairment, or M.C.I., a type of memory impairment that is often a precursor of Alzheimer's disease (Bakalar, 2019, para.1).

Builds Stronger and Healthier Bones.

Dairy products like milk are usually the ones known for improving your bone health. However, this benefit is also surprisingly peculiar to broccoli because it contains high levels of both calcium and vitamin K. Vitamin K is an essential nutrient needed to improve our bone health in general. With calcium and other nutrients like magnesium, zinc, and phosphorus, Vitamin K also plays an important role in increasing bone mineral density and reducing fracture rates in those with osteoporosis. It also aids in blood clotting. Since broccoli is rich in this nutrient, you can easily increase your bone density by consuming Vitamin K and Calcium through your diet.

Though you might not believe this, onions have also been discovered to be very effective in boosting bone density, decreasing bone loss, and preventing osteoporosis, especially in elderly persons (Kubala, 2018, para.11). A study conducted with 507 perimenopausal and postmenopausal women found that those who ate onions at least once a day had a 5% greater overall bone density than individuals who ate them once a month or less. The study also revealed that older women who most frequently ate onions decreased their risk of hip fracture by more than 20% compared to those who never ate them.

Improves Eye Health

Broccoli contains a measurable amount of antioxidants, Lutein and Zeaxanthin, as well as beta-carotene. All these rich nutrients are great for eye health as they help protect the eyes against macular degeneration and cataract. They also prevent oxidative stress and cellular damage in your eyes. Though many of us don't realize this, we tend to slowly damage our eyes with the harmful radiation from continued use of gadgets like cell phones and computer screens. Fortunately for us, consuming broccoli can help in repairing and reducing those damages. Broccoli also helps in lowering the risk of night blindness. This condition is mostly associated with a deficiency of vitamin A. Broccoli provides us with beta-carotene, which is converted into vitamin A.

How to Include these Superfoods in Your Meals

Mushroom

Before we even discuss how you can incorporate mushrooms into your diet, make sure to always select and buy only fresh mushrooms, those that are firm, dry, and unbruised. Completely avoid mushrooms that appear slimy or withered. Essentially, you must ensure that you buy from a reliable source, most likely a grocery or health food store.

In terms of proper storage, you can keep your mushrooms in a paper bag inside the refrigerator for up to five days. Just make sure you don't wash or trim them until it is time to cook with them. Now, regarding cooking, here is how you can make it work with mushrooms:

1. Cook any type of mushroom with onions or garlic and butter for a quick, tasty side dish.

2. Add sliced mushrooms to stir-fries.

3. Sprinkle and top your salad with raw, sliced cremini or white mushrooms.

4. Add them as an ingredient in homemade pizza, breakfast scrambles, and quiches.

5. You can also try removing the stems of portobello mushrooms, marinating the caps in a mixture of olive oil, onion, garlic, and vinegar for 1 hour, then grilling them for 10 minutes.

6. Grilled mushrooms taste great when added to sandwiches or wraps

7. Mix mushrooms into cooked beef, chicken, or turkey.

8. Use mushrooms as an ingredient in pasta sauce.

Broccoli

1. To buy high-quality broccoli, always go for the ones with unblemished, dark green tops and firm stalks with no soft spots. Note that this versatile vegetable can be steamed, fried, boiled, and roasted.

2. Oven-roast your broccoli and use them as a topping for your pasta dishes or grain salads.

3. Squeeze fresh lemon juice over roasted broccoli or drizzle it with a tangy sauce.

4. Use chopped broccoli florets to make broccoli salad, and serve with a creamy dressing and anything grilled.

5. Grill your broccoli and season it lightly with a drizzle of olive oil and a splash of lemon juice

Onions

Remember we briefly discussed onions having a reputation for making people cry during the cutting or chopping process and how many people tend to make assumptions that this superfood improves eye health because of this reason? Well, firstly, you should understand this response occurs due to the presence of a chemical called syn-Propanethial-S-oxide. Actually, this gas is a compound liquid that acts as a lachrymatory agent, meaning that it causes tears or stings the eyes. It really has nothing to do with improving eyesight.

In case you are unaware, there is a way you can reduce the tears during chopping. The National Onion Association recommends chilling an onion for 30 minutes then cutting off its top. Afterward, you should peel the onion's outer layer and leave the root intact, as this part has the highest concentration of lachrymatory agents.

Onions are a staple in many kitchens. This is because no ingredient is quite like it when adding subtle sweetness and bolstering other flavors simultaneously. This culinary luxury can be roasted, grilled, pickled, caramelized, battered, or deep-fried. Now here is how you can use it in your meals.

1. Obviously, your stir-fry dishes cannot be completed with you throwing in some chopped onions.
2. Caramelize your onions and add them when baking savory loaves of bread or cakes.
3. Use onions as a base for your soups, stocks, and sauces,
4. Top your salads or tacos with chopped raw onions.
5. You can also use it to fill your sandwich.
6. Try adding cooked onions to omelets, frittatas, or quiches.
7. Toss them in when roasting your chicken, turkey, or meat.
8. For a tasty homemade salad dressing. You can also blend raw onions with fresh herbs, vinegar, and olive oil.
9. Prepare a homemade salsa with onions, tomatoes, and fresh cilantro.

7

CINNAMON, GINGER, AND NUTMEG

This chapter will explore the three fall spices that really deserve a special place in your kitchen and life. And maybe they are all right there in your kitchen, but you just never knew how much of an essential medicine each of them is! If that's the case, then read on.

Generally, it is well-known that whether they are used individually or are well-combined, cinnamon, ginger, and nutmeg can inject exciting variety and flavor into the classic recipes and even your own homemade creations. But far beyond that, these superfoods can offer magical benefits just like medicines.

Let's start with our favorite household spice, cinnamon. Blessed with a unique, pleasant flavor and warm smell, the cinnamon spice is obtained from a small evergreen tree's inner bark. The bark is peeled and laid in the sun to dry, where it curls up into rolls which is what we call cinnamon sticks. Then these sticks can be ground to form cinnamon powder. You see, cinnamon has been used as both a culinary ingredient and a curing agent throughout history, dating back as far as

Ancient Egypt. Can you believe that this superfood was once traded as a currency and a gift fit only for kings? Quite rare and valuable, isn't it? Good thing for us it is now cheap and available in almost all supermarkets. Interestingly, this still doesn't depreciate the fact that cinnamon has medicinal properties that can create a powerful effect on our health. Have you ever wondered the source of that distinct smell and flavor of cinnamon? The fragrance and taste result from the oily part of the cinnamon, which is very high in the fragrant compound cinnamaldehyde. Some scientists believe that this compound is also responsible for most of cinnamon's powerful health benefits.

Closely related to cinnamon is another one of the healthiest spices on the planet, Ginger. It also has a unique fragrance and flavor thanks to its natural oils, with the most important one being gingerol. Though ginger is a flowering plant that originated in Southeast Asia, it has been added as an essential ingredient in almost all culinary dishes in many traditional cultures worldwide due to its numerous healing capabilities. Even with over 3000 years of rich history, ginger has never changed in its medicinal properties. True to its title of being a superfood, ginger has anti-inflammatory, antibacterial, antiviral, and other healthful properties that can thwart off health problems.

The spiced superfood, Nutmeg, is a popular spice from the seeds of Myristica fragrans, a tropical evergreen tree native to Indonesia. And just so you know, Indonesia produces the majority of the world's nutmeg. Nutmeg has a warm, slightly nutty flavor that does wonders when added to many dishes, both savory and sweet. Obviously, it is only for this reason that most of us make use of nutmeg. What you may not know is that this superfood contains an impressive array of powerful nutrients and compounds that may help prevent various diseases and promote your overall health.

Nutritional Breakdown of Cinnamon, Ginger, the essential and Nutmeg

What are the exact nutrients contained in these three fall superfoods? Below is the nutritional breakdown of nutrients in 1 teaspoon (tsp) of ground cinnamon:

Calories	6
Carbohydrates	2 g
Dietary fiber	1 g (4 percent daily value, or DV)
Calcium	26 mg (2.6 percent DV)
Potassium	11 mg (0.23 percent DV)
Magnesium	2 mg (0.5 percent DV)
Phosphorus	2 mg (0.2 percent DV)
Vitamin K	1 microgram (1.22 percent DV)
Vitamin A	8 international units (0.16 percent DV)

Next, 1 tablespoon of fresh ginger contains:

Calories	4.8
Carbohydrate	1.07 grams
Dietary fiber	12 grams
Protein	11 grams
Fat	0.5 grams
Sugar	1 gram
Potassium	8.3 grams
Calcium	0.32mg

Finally, 1 teaspoon serving of nutmeg contains:

Calories	12
Protein	0.13 grams
Fat	0.8 grams
Carbohydrates	1.08 grams
Fiber	0.46 grams
Sugar	1 gram
Phosphorus	4.69 mg
Magnesium	4.03 mg

Calcium	4.05 mg

Health Benefits of Cinnamon, Ginger, and Nutmeg

Lower Blood Sugars

Cinnamon is a superfood equipped with various effective mechanisms for lowering blood sugar. Firstly, cinnamon can reduce insulin resistance, a condition that is common with type-2 diabetes patients. Insulin is one of the essential hormones responsible for transporting blood sugar from your bloodstream to your cells. However, a diabetic condition causes the body to become resistant to the effects of this hormone. However, by consuming the right amount of cinnamon, you can help increase insulin sensitivity and allow this important hormone to do its job, which will, in turn, lower blood sugar levels.

Another anti-diabetic mechanism that cinnamon uses is to decrease the amount of glucose that enters your bloodstream after eating is by simply interfering with different digestive enzymes, which slow the breakdown of carbohydrates in your digestive tract. Interestingly, a compound in cinnamon can mimic insulin, though it acts much slower than the insulin itself. This compound acts on the cells and greatly improves their glucose uptake (Leech, 2018, para.5)

A relatively new area of research has found that ginger also has powerful anti-diabetic properties. The study, which involved 41 participants with type 2 diabetes, revealed that consuming 2 grams of ginger powder per day reduced fasting blood sugar by 12%. It also improved hemoglobin A1c (HbA1c). HbA1c was reduced by 10% over a period of 12 weeks. (Leech, 2018, para. 6). The report also showed that ginger improves the various heart disease risk factors in people with type 2 diabetes. The antioxidant content in nutmeg may also help prevent your blood sugar level from spiking and enhances pancreatic function.

Helps in Managing Neurodegenerative Diseases

We all know the term "Neuro" kind of has something to do with the brain, right? Neurodegenerative diseases are conditions often characterized by a progressive reduction in brain cell structure or function. Alzheimer's is one of the most common types, and in the previous chapter, we discussed how the buildup of a protein called "tau" in the brain is a prominent hallmark. The good news is that two compounds found in cinnamon also appear to inhibit this protein's buildup.

The anti-inflammatory properties available in ginger are also believed to be effective in improving good brain functionality. A study by Evidence-Based Complementary and Alternative Medicine determined that ginger root could increase the presence of mind and our cognitive function.

How about Nutmeg? Well, this spice does not only really help in managing neurodegenerative diseases, it also works as an aphrodisiac. This implies that the chemicals in this spice can stimulate the nerve cells in your brain, causing the release of the feel-good hormones into the body. By doing so, nutmeg can improve your mood and give you a calming effect.

Aids in Indigestion

Indigestion is a condition that is often characterized by re-emerging pain and severe discomfort in the upper part of your stomach when it is unable to empty itself. Taking ginger can help empty your stomach faster and treat or prevent indigestion. Sometimes, certain gases form in the intestinal tract during digestion. The enzymes in ginger can help the body break up and expel this gas, providing relief from any discomfort. Some researchers also revealed that ginger might have beneficial effects on trypsin and pancreatic lipase, the two enzymes that are important for digestion.

Furthermore, cinnamon and nutmeg are also known to have medicinal properties that can ease digestive discomfort though they may not be quite as effective as ginger.

Helps in Relieving Nausea and Morning Sickness

Ginger, particularly, has been proven to be highly effective in alleviating morning sickness and relieving nausea. If you have a vomiting sensation or are suffering from nausea due to motion sickness, then you can use ginger as a natural home remedy to treat it. This superfood appears to be the most effective when it comes to pregnancy-related nausea, especially morning sickness. According to a review of 12 studies that included 1,278 pregnant women, 1.1–1.5 grams of ginger can significantly reduce nausea symptoms (Leech, 2020, para. 4).

However, though ginger is scientifically safe for pregnant women, ensure that you consult your doctor before taking large amounts. It is highly recommended that pregnant women close to labor or who've had miscarriages avoid ginger.

Reduces Menstrual Cramps

Traditionally, ginger helps relieve different pain types, including the pain that a woman goes through during her menstrual cycle. Oftentimes, this pain can be unbearable for some women. Some studies have recommended that taking 1 gram of ginger a day can ease the pain menstrual cycle if taken for 3 days. In fact, more recent studies have also concluded that ginger is equally as effective as drugs such as mefenamic acid and acetaminophen/caffeine/ibuprofen, which are well-known for being menstrual pain relief drugs. Essentially, this makes using ginger a much safer option to avoid the side-effects that medicated drugs can offer.

Helps in Treating Osteoarthritis

Osteoarthritis is a condition commonly found among most older people. The symptoms majorly include severe pain and stiffness in the joints. Ginger, nutmeg and cinnamon, all consist of anti-inflammatory components and antioxidants that can reduce swelling, inflammation, joint pain, muscle spasms, and other symptoms associated with this condition.

Helps in Managing Dental Problems

Toothaches, bad breath, cavities, and other gum diseases are usually caused by bacteria like Streptococcus mutans and Aggregatibacter actinomycetemcomitans. Nutmeg is well-known for having antibacterial and antimicrobial properties. In fact, you will find that nutmeg oil is mostly used as an ingredient in many of your dental products at home. This is because the spice's antibacterial properties have proven to be particularly effective against the oral pathogens that cause dental infections and bad breath.

Eugenol, one of the essential oils in nutmeg, plays a great role in relieving toothaches. Another chemical found in nutmeg, Macelignan, can also help prevent cavities.

Now the benefits of relieving dental infections are not only limited to nutmeg. Cinnamaldehyde, one of the main active components of cinnamon, and its other antimicrobial components may also help prevent tooth decay and reduce bad breath.

Reduces Insomnia

Nutmeg is another superfood that can improve your sleep, both in duration and quality. Mixing a little nutmeg in a glass full of milk has been an age-old tradition passed on for generations. Consuming this superfood is an organic and healthy way of inducing sleep and treating insomnia. As a mother, if you haven't tried it yet, you can also give your children warm milk with a little bit of nutmeg powder mixed in it before they go to sleep. You may find that the duration and quality of sleeping improves.

How to Include these Superfoods in Your Meals

Cinnamon

The best way to store your cinnamon is to keep it in an airtight container in a dark place. Cinnamon sticks can last for about a year, but ground cinnamon may start to lose flavor after a few months of storage. No doubt, this popular ancient spice has a great power to evoke a degree of nostalgia and luxury in our dishes. Here are methods you can use to experience this feeling!

1. You may mix cinnamon with sugar and sprinkle it on toast or atop a steaming pumpkin spice latte.
2. Drop a pinch of ground cinnamon into a hot wintertime cider or feature it when baking an aromatic, fresh apple pie.
3. Add cinnamon to drinks such as fruit smoothies or turmeric lattes.
4. Sprinkle over almonds and roast them in the oven.
5. Mix in Greek yogurt as a snack.

Ginger

Adding ginger to your diet is a wise health choice; it can also add a savory and spicy kick to your meals. Here are a few ways to do it:

1. Use it to make ginger tea from scratch adding other ingredients like honey, sugar, or even lime.
2. If you're not a fan of ginger tea, then sprinkle a little bit of freshly grated ginger root into your favorite tea for an added kick.
3. Add ginger to your smoothies to make them more packed with health benefits.
4. Ginger pairs well with fish, so you can use it to season your seafood.
5. Create a ginger marinade by using pepper, salt, cloves, thyme with chicken or salmon.
6. Use ginger to add flavor when cooking chicken broth. Or just make ginger soup.
7. Tiny pieces of ginger can also work as topping for your homemade chicken pizza.
8. Sprinkle small chopped pieces of ginger to ramp up your stir-fry.

Nutmeg

You can use both ground and whole nutmeg in your dishes and

drinks. But if you're using a whole nutmeg, grate it with a Microplane or grater with smaller holes. Now, the first rule you must learn when cooking with nutmeg is that a little does a lot. So, you should never consume more than is ordinarily required for your food preparation. Failing to adhere to this rule can be highly toxic and even fatal. Now how do we use nutmeg to spice up our meals?

1. Add it when making either warm or cold beverages, such as apple cider, hot chocolate, chai tea, turmeric lattes, and smoothies.
2. Sprinkle the spice when cooking savory, meat-based dishes, such as pork chops and lamb curry.
3. You can add nutmeg to spice up your creamy sauces and cheesy dishes, such as bechamel, alfredo sauce, and soufflés.
4. Nutmeg is a key ingredient in many baked goods like bread, cake, cookies. So, bake with it!
5. To create a deep, interesting flavor, add them in desserts like pumpkin pie, custards, and eggnog.
6. Use it to season starchy vegetables like sweet potatoes, butternut squash, and pumpkin.

8

SALMON AND TURKEY

Taking a quick flashback to our first chapter, you would remember that we stated that though most superfoods are plant-based, a few of them belong to the fish and poultry family! This chapter will focus on salmon and turkey, two of the most nutritionally dense foods in this category of uncommon superfoods.

Salmon is one of the most loved and commonly consumed fish, thanks to its versatile nature and excellent taste. You know, it is that kind of food that tastes great at all hours of the day, be it breakfast, brunch, or dinner. Another good feature of this fatty fish is that it is widely available for consumption in many cultures worldwide. There are several types of salmon found in the northern Atlantic and Pacific oceans. Now the big question is, "Is Salmon healthy enough to be a superfood?" This is a fair question to ask since it is well-known that salmon is an oily fish with a rich amount of fats. But rest assured that the fat it contains is completely healthy, and you will confirm that as you read further!

There are so many reasons that salmon should be an important part of your diet. The most prominent of them is that it is one of the most nutritious foods on the planet. But like the usual, we don't make claims without supporting them with science-backed evidence. This popular fatty fish is an excellent food source with a wide range of essential nutrients and health benefits that can reduce risk factors for several diseases. It is highly praised for its high protein content and omega-3 fatty acids. We will discuss more of this when we explore its nutritional breakdown and health benefits.

Nevertheless, it is worth it for you to understand that wild salmon contains more nutritional value than the farmed ones. Now, what's the difference? The farmed salmon are raised and fed based on an artificial pellet-based diet, but the wild salmon are raised based on their natural diet consisting of crustaceans, flies, and smaller fishes which they can easily find in the wild. Now, we are not saying that eating salmon from a hatchery is not nutritious. That will be utterly wrong since they may be the ones that are more widely available. However, the point is that the wild-caught salmon has a little more nutritional value.

On to the turkey! Did you know that Benjamin Franklin once referred to the large bird as "respectable" and a "Bird of Courage"? Guess that it explains why it is always the main course or staple food on everybody's mind during the holidays. Come on, let's ask ourselves, "What's a holiday feast without a roasted turkey?" Incomplete!

Apart from its high demand during festive periods, this popular holiday food is highly rich in protein, vitamins, and minerals, all of which have a specific range of health benefits associated with them. Just like Salmon, turkeys can be hunted in the wild, as well as raised on farms. Now let's do a breakdown of these two superfoods' impressive nutritional profiles, after which we will take an in-depth look at their possible health benefits.

Nutritional Breakdown of Salmon and Turkey

According to the USDA National Nutrient Database, 3 ounces (oz) which are approximately 85 grams (g) of cooked Atlantic salmon, is packed with the following nutrients:

Calories	175	Phosphorus	23% of RDA
Fat	10.5 grams	Thiamin	12% of RDA
Carbohydrate	0 grams	Vitamin A	4% of RDA
Protein	18.79 grams		
Vitamin B12	82% of (RDA)		
Selenium	46 % of RDA		
Niacin	28 % of RDA		

Turkey - Two thick slices (84 grams) of turkey contain

Calories	117	Zinc	12% of the DV
Protein	24 grams	Sodium	26% of the DV
Fat	2 grams	Phosphorous	28% of the DV
Carbs	0 grams	Choline	12% of the DV
Niacin (vitamin B3)	61% of the Daily Value (DV)	Magnesium	6% of the DV
Vitamin B6	49% of the DV	Potassium	4% of the DV
Vitamin B12	29% of the DV		
Selenium	46% of the DV		

Note that the nutrients contained in your turkey depend on the cut. For example, dark meat, which is usually found in its active muscles like the legs or thighs, tends to have more fat and calories than white meat. White meat tends to contain slightly more protein. Another thing worthy to note is that turkey skin is high in fat. This means that meat cuts with the skin on will have more calories and fat than skinless cuts.

Health Benefits of Salmon and Turkey

Offers a Loaded Amount of Protein

Consuming the right amount of salmon and turkey is really an efficient way to get in all the amino acids that your body requires. Just about three ounces of each of these two superfoods offer you between 18 to 24 grams of proteins. That's quite a lot, isn't it? And we all know that the importance of consuming protein-rich foods cannot be overemphasized.

Protein is essential for maintaining our tissues and muscle mass. It also acts as chemical messengers, transporting nutrients around the body. Some proteins' fibrous nature also helps structure-specific cells and tissues by providing them with stiffness and rigidity. It also helps form antibodies to fight invading infections. High levels of protein can help regulate insulin levels and actually combat fatigue.

Apart from these few benefits we just stated, there are so many other benefits of proteins. Thus, by seeing just how essential these nutrients are, you will agree that your diet should include salmon and turkey.

Lowers Risk of Heart Diseases.

Salmon is a rich source of omega-3 fatty acids (EPA and DHA) and potassium. Two prominent nutrients contribute greatly to our heart health. Like we stated earlier, the fats contained in salmon are the good kind. They help in reducing artery inflammation, lowering cholesterol levels, and maintaining blood pressure levels. The rich potassium content in salmon also helps to control your blood pressure and prevent excess fluid retention. You see that pinkish-red color for which salmon is well known? It has some added benefits here. That hue comes from an antioxidant called astaxanthin. This antioxidant helps decrease bad cholesterol and increase the good.

When combined, the activities of these nutrients significantly reduce heart-related medical problems like heart attacks, strokes, arrhythmia, high blood pressure, and high triglycerides.

Aids in Decreasing Risk of Cancer

Another impressive benefit of salmon is that its omega-3 fatty acid content has been medically proven to profoundly affect the cells of certain cancers such as skin cancer, prostate cancer, colorectal cancer, liver cancer, and UVB-induced skin cancer. The tumors associated with the aforementioned cancerous conditions can be treated and prevented with omega-3 fatty acids.

Turkey is also blessed with anti-cancer properties, thanks to its rich source of the trace mineral, selenium. Scientific studies have suggested that selenium intake can reduce the incidence of cancer. Besides its cancer-fighting properties, selenium also helps your body produce thyroid hormones, regulating your metabolism and growth rate. (O'Brien, 2019, para. 7)

Perhaps, the next time you plan to use red meat for your cooking, you should consider using turkey or salmon instead. This is because they are healthy alternatives, unlike red meat, which some observational studies have linked to an increased risk of colon cancer and heart diseases.

Promotes Sleep and Boosts your Mood.

Turkey meat contains tryptophan, the hormone that promotes sleep. According to the Australian Turkey Federation, the tryptophan present in turkey meat effectively treats chronic insomnia. Beyond aiding sleep, scientific evidence also suggests that tryptophan plays a significant role in strengthening the immune system. This is quite justifiable since we all know that getting good sleep helps boost your immune system.

Now, coming from the fact that it is a festive-holiday food, you shouldn't be surprised to see that turkey has mood-enhancing properties. The body also uses the tryptophan hormone to make serotonin, a neurotransmitter that helps improve your mood.

Helps with Weight Loss

Salmon is a low-calorie food that takes a lot of energy and calories to digest slower. It makes you feel full longer, thereby reducing your appetite and making weight loss easier. Though it seems quite ironic that a fatty fish will help with weight loss, the fat content in salmon is mostly good and doesn't make you gain weight. If your assumptions about its fatty nature were a problem before, then by now, you should be convinced that it is absolutely healthy and advisable to include salmon in your diet plan.

Great for Skin and Hair

Thanks to its carotenoid antioxidants of astaxanthin, salmon effectively keeps our skin healthy and increases our hair growth. The antioxidant can help combat the signs of UV damage and prevent water loss. It sounds like what sunscreen will do, right?

This antioxidant doesn't work in isolation. Instead, it works in collaboration with the Omega-3 fatty acids as well as vitamins. Together, they improve your skin quality and health. These nutrients also tremendously reduce free radical damage that is responsible for aging. So simply put, salmon benefits your skin and hair with its anti-aging benefits.

Promotes Brain Health

You must have heard somewhere that fish is 'brain food.' Well, there is convincing evidence to support this claim. Studies suggest that the high presence of omega-3 fatty acids in the fish reduces age-related brain problems like Alzheimer's disease, depression, multiple sclerosis, dementia. The high levels of omega-3 fatty acids basically work in association with the vitamin A, vitamin D, and selenium in salmon to boost brain function and improve memory. Eating salmon during pregnancy can even result in improved fetal brain development and health. Recently, researchers found that the consumption of many of the nutrients found in salmon is connected to a lower risk of affective disorders, such as depression. (Butler, 2017, Para.11)

How to Include these Superfoods in your Meals

Salmon

Never forget that in terms of quality, wild-caught salmon is your best bet! Here are some quick, tasty tips on how you can work more salmon into your diet:

1. Add simply cooked salmon to your pasta or rice dishes.
2. Roast or grill your salmon, season it with salt and pepper and serve with a lemon-yogurt sauce.
3. Make a creamy salmon stew.
4. Make classic salmon cakes by blending the fish with mashed or cooked chopped potatoes.
5. Use salmon herbs and seasoning to make salmon burgers.
6. Treat your salmon like beef and make a red wine sauce with thyme and balsamic vinegar or with beef stock and mushrooms to go with it.

Turkey

Completely avoid or perhaps limit to a large extent your intake of processed turkey products, such as turkey bacon, hot dogs, sausages, and sandwich meat. Even when frozen, these products are high in sodium due to the added salt and preservatives, which they are continuously injected with, to extend their shelf life and cut costs.

Thus, it is in your best interest to always go for fresh, lean, organic, and pasture-raised turkey. These kinds are usually raised in humane conditions, with free access to nature and without being injected with antibiotics. Aside from this, their meat is usually healthier and more flavorful.

Turkey meat is often roasted in the oven, but you can also use a slow-cooker or crockpot to slow-cook it until tender. Make sure to cook the turkey until the internal temperature reaches 165° Fahrenheit to reduce foodborne illness risk. You can include turkey in your diet in endless ways. Some of them include:

1. Give your salad a good protein boost by adding roasted turkey, whether hot or cold.
2. Turkey meat can make your soup taste way better.
3. Use turkey when making curries instead of using chicken.
4. Turkey meats also work perfectly in casseroles.
5. Combine turkey meat with your favorite toppings and spreads, such as lettuce, tomato, mustard, or pesto.
6. You can also make your stock from turkey bones.
7. Make burger patties by mixing ground turkey with breadcrumbs.
8. Used minced turkey meat to replace ground beef in dishes like spaghetti Bolognese or cottage pie.
9. If you are trying to keep your fat intake in check, then stick to white turkey meat. You can bake, broil or sauté it in as little oil as possible, using broth, lemon, or orange juice as a basting sauce.

9

SWEET POTATO

Our nutritional all-star and superfood of this chapter is the popular delicious root vegetable, sweet potato, also known as the Ipomoea batatas. They are grown across different parts of the world in a variety of sizes and colors. In terms of color, most sweet potatoes are usually orange, but others come in purple, yellow, white, pink, and red. Sweet potatoes offer naturally sweet and creamy tastes whether it is boiled, baked, or fried.

This root vegetable is tasty and colorful, but is also a powerhouse of numerous nutrients packed with medicinal benefits. Some of us might doubt the validity of this claim, and honestly, you are not wrong to have that thought considering the very name of this superfood suggests that they're loaded with too much sugar-and-starch. However, in due time you will totally believe that sweet potatoes are a nutritious gem; keep reading!

Most of us tend to interchange the terms "sweet potato" and "yam" for each other. However, the two foods are not the same in any way.

Yams have a drier texture and a starchier content than sweet potatoes. Even "potatoes" and "sweet potatoes" are not actually related. They may both be called 'potatoes,' but botanically, the sweet potato belongs to the bindweed or morning glory family, which is different from the nightshade family where the white potato sits.

Nutritional Breakdown of Sweet Potato

One cup (200 grams) of baked sweet potato with skin provides the following nutrients:

Calories	180	Vitamin C	65% of the DV
Carbs	41.4 grams	Manganese	50% of the DV
Protein	4 grams	Vitamin B6	29% of the DV
Fat	0.3 grams	Potassium	27% of the DV
Fiber	6.6 grams	Pantothenic acid	18% of the DV
Vitamin A	69% of the Daily Value (DV)	Copper	16% of the DV

In addition to these nutrients, sweet potatoes, especially the orange and purple varieties, are a rich source of antioxidants that protect your body from free radicals.

Health Benefits of Sweet Potato

Helps in Managing and Lowering Risk of Type-2 Diabetes.
The assumption that some of us tend to have about sweet potatoes being too starchy for our health is wrong based on some science-backed evidence. How is that? Studies have found that people who

consume more fiber appear to have a lower risk of developing type 2 diabetes. (Ware, 2019, para.3). One cup of baked sweet potato provides about 6 grams of fiber, which is more than a quarter of the daily recommended minimum. Thus, the high fiber content in sweet potatoes makes them a slow-burning starch which implies that they won't spike your blood sugar and insulin levels. Ironically, 77% of the fiber in sweet potatoes is insoluble, and these insoluble fibers play a significant role in the fight against diabetes. This kind of fiber helps a lot in promoting insulin sensitivity in diabetic patients. By doing so, they can regulate the amount of sugar in the blood. The remaining 10% to 15% fiber soluble effectively reduces food consumption and spikes in blood sugar.

Another vital nutrient shown and proven to minimize the risk of individuals developing type II diabetes is magnesium. Fortunately, you can get a good amount of it by consuming sweet potatoes.

Reduces Risk of Cancer

Sweet potatoes offer various antioxidants, which may have anti-cancer fighting properties. They are an excellent beta-carotene source; a plant pigments whose body converts into the vitamin's active form. Apart from being pro-vitamin, beta-carotene is also a powerful antioxidant that can prevent cellular damage, mainly caused by unstable molecules called free radicals. High levels of free radicals in the body mean more cellular damage, increasing the risk of certain cancers like lung cancer. Essentially, beta-carotene reduces the oxidation process and may provide potential protection from such types of cancer.

Another group of antioxidants found explicitly in purple sweet potatoes, anthocyanins, have been shown to slow the growth of certain types of cancer cells, including those of the bladder, colon, stomach, and breast. Some studies have suggested that the antioxidants are primarily found in the peel of sweet potatoes, in particular. Thus, to get the most nutrition from your sweet potatoes, eat them with the skin!

Helps Regulate Blood Pressure Levels

Sweet potatoes can help control your blood pressure levels because they contain rich amounts of magnesium and potassium, both of which play an essential role in regulating blood pressure. One cup of sweet potato baked in its skin offers about 950 mg of potassium which is twice the amount you will get from consuming a medium banana.

Studies have shown that a higher intake of potassium results in a reduction in blood pressure, which significantly decreases the risk of developing a stroke or any other heart-related problem. But how is it possible that potassium can be this effective?

The nutrient essentially flushes excess sodium and fluid out of your body, lowers blood pressure, and reduces strain on the heart. It also helps regulate the heart rhythm and muscle contractions.

High blood pressure is the dominant risk factor for hypertension. Fortunately, magnesium is a dietary component that is considered effective in preventing and reducing hypertension. Most people don't know is that a magnesium deficiency in the body increases the risk factors for the development of hypertension and some other cardiovascular diseases. But including sweet potatoes in your diet is one of the most effective ways to supply your body with its required amount of magnesium.

Helps Improve Digestion

By now, we should know that foods that are high in fiber help promote a healthy digestive system. By being fiber-high, sweet potatoes are also not an exception. This superfood has a sufficient amount of both soluble and insoluble fiber contained in them. Since your body cannot digest either of them, the soluble and insoluble fiber stays within your digestive tract and provides various health benefits.

The soluble fiber usually absorbs water and softens your stool, while the insoluble fibers add bulk to your stool. They don't absorb water. By performing these responsibilities mentioned above, the fibers help prevent constipation and promote regularity for a healthy digestive tract.

The antioxidants in sweet potatoes have also been very effective in providing great benefits to the digestive system. Some studies found the antioxidants in purple sweet potatoes, anthocyanins promote healthy gut bacteria growth, including certain bacteria like Bifidobacterium and Lactobacillus species. The amounts of these types of bacteria within the intestines are linked with better digestive health and a lower risk of conditions like irritable bowel syndrome (IBS) and infectious diarrhea (Julson, 2019, para.6)

Promotes Healthy Vision

Food & Nutrition Research has shown that the anthocyanins in purple sweet potatoes are beneficial to the eyes. They help protect the eye cells from damage, and this responsibility is of great significance to your overall eye health.

Beta-carotene has also been found to be great in supporting healthy eyesight. This antioxidant, which is usually found in orange-fleshed sweet potatoes, is responsible for the vegetable's bright orange hue. When consumed, the antioxidant converts to vitamin A in your body and is used to create light-detecting receptors inside your eyes. Eating such food may help prevent a special type of blindness known as xerophthalmia, which is linked to a deficiency in vitamin A.

Reduces Inflammation

When low-grade inflammation remains unchecked and untreated, it raises the risk of nearly every chronic disease, including obesity, type 2 diabetes, heart disease, and cancer. However, the presence of natural anti-inflammatory compounds in sweet potatoes makes the root vegetables an essential superfood for preventing and reducing chronic inflammation in the body, especially at the cellular level.

Some studies have indicated that antioxidant anthocyanins in the purple sweet potato are essential in reducing and preventing inflammation, especially in colon cancer cells. Another research on animals has shown reduced inflammation in brain tissue and nerve tissue after consuming purple sweet potatoes.

Another anti-inflammatory property of sweet potatoes is their high concentration of choline. Choline is a versatile nutrient that can reduce and restrain inflammatory responses in the body, resulting in less inflammation. Studies on animal models have confirmed this claim.

Apart from these two compounds, sweet potatoes also contain a significant number of vitamins, most of which have powerful anti-inflammatory properties. These vitamins have the power to inhibit the production of active inflammatory components in the body. This means that by consuming sweet potatoes, your body is provided with the services of three whole anti-inflammatory components in just one go!

Strengthen your Immune System

If you have properly studied the nutritional breakdown above, then you will realize that just a cup of baked sweet potato can offer you more than half of your daily vitamin C needs. Consuming the same portion also supplies 69% of your recommended daily intake of vitamin A! These two nutrients are vital for supporting and strengthening your immune function, which is especially important during cold and flu season. Interestingly, orange-fleshed sweet potatoes are actually one of the richest natural sources of beta-carotene, containing a higher content than carrots.

Helps Boost Fertility

For this chapter, we saved the best for the last! Obviously, this particular health benefit may come as a surprise to most people. Nevertheless, sweet potatoes contain a good amount of iron which is a crucial mineral for promoting fertility in women of childbearing age. In fact, studies have found that anemia or iron deficiency can be a major cause of infertility among women. Thus, increasing dietary intake of iron may enable women to conceive a few months to a year after the treatment. The presence of dietary iron in sweet potatoes also reduces the risk of ovulatory infertility.

How to Include Sweet Potato in Your Meals

When trying to select the sweet potatoes for your home-made meals, it is important to check that the potato is firm with smooth, taut skin. In terms of storage, put them in a cool, dry place. Just make sure they are not in storage for more than 3-5 weeks. Also, always keep in mind that eating a sweet potato with its skin can increase your most likely nutritional value. In case you aren't sure how to use sweet potatoes as savory additions to your meals, here are some helpful tips!

1. Roast sweet potatoes to bring out their natural flavor and add them to your garden salad, topping it with balsamic vinegar.
2. Add roasted sweet potatoes to pancakes.
3. Bake them and drizzle with a combo of ground cinnamon and maple syrup thinned with a bit of warm water.
4. Use them as a base for your soups after pureeing them with low-sodium organic veggie broth.
5. Oven-bake or fry your thinly sliced sweet potatoes to satisfy your French fry craving.
6. Make a toast with your sweet potatoes by cutting them into thin slices, toasting them, and topping them with nut butter or avocado ingredients.
7. Boil and mash your sweet potatoes with milk and seasoning, then use it as a fantastic addition to desserts such as no-bake cookies, brownies, overnight oats, or even sweet potato pie.
8. You can even whip them into a smoothie.

10

AVOCADOS

Originated in southern Mexico and Columbia about 7,000 years ago, avocados have earned a special place in the kitchens and hearts of their lovers. This nutritionally-dense superfood varies in shape and color — from pear-shaped to round and from green to black. But the most common one that you would most likely find in the grocery stores around you are the Hass avocado. This common variety is characterized by a green, scale-like skin and pear shape, which earned it the name "Alligator pear."

Though many people tend to label avocado as a vegetable, it is botanically considered a berry because of its fleshy pulp and sizable single seed. Avocados are a little more expensive than the fruits we have discussed earlier. This doesn't seem to affect their popularity, perhaps due to its rich, creamy texture and mild flavor.

Apart from their unique taste and texture, avocados are super nutritious. They contain about 20 different vitamins and minerals. Did you just say "wow!"? Of course, you should; that is a wide variety of nutrients. Another super quality of avocados is that they are the only fruit that provides a substantial amount of healthy monounsaturated fatty acids (MUFA). Now, this is something to get us more curious, so let's quickly break down their nutritional profile and then explore the specific health benefits you can get from consuming this fruit.

Nutritional Breakdown of Avocados

Calories	160	Vitamin C	17% of the DV
Protein	2 grams	Potassium	14% of the DV
Fats	15 grams	Vitamin B5	14% of the DV
Carbs	9 grams	Vitamin B6	13% of the DV
Fiber	7 grams	Vitamin E	10% of the DV
Vitamin K	26% of the daily value (DV)		
Folate	20% of the DV		

Avocado also contains small amounts of magnesium, manganese, copper, iron, zinc, phosphorus, and vitamins A, B1 (thiamine), B2 (riboflavin), and B3 (niacin).

Health Benefits of Avocados

Improves your Heart Health
Numerous studies have proven that eating avocado can eliminate different heart disease risk factors such as "bad" LDL cholesterol and

blood triglycerides. But these benefits don't happen like magic; avocados are excellent sources of potassium, folate, and fiber, all of which can strengthen the health of your heart and cardiovascular system. Starting with potassium, this is a nutrient that most of us don't get enough of. However, avocado supplies the body with an even higher potassium content than a banana which is considered a typically potassium-high food. So, what use is this nutrient to your heart? As we learned in the previous chapters, having a high potassium intake helps support healthy blood pressure levels, reducing the risk of chronic heart conditions like heart attacks, hypertension, and strokes.

Furthermore, avocados are one of the fattiest plant-based foods in existence, but most of the fat contained in them is oleic acid, a monounsaturated fatty acid. Some research has shown that this heart-healthy fatty acid can significantly reduce total cholesterol levels, blood triglycerides, and cardiovascular inflammation by consuming avocados regularly.

Avocados also contain a natural plant sterol called beta-sitosterol. Studies have proven that the regular consumption of beta-sitosterol and other plant sterols can help maintain healthy cholesterol levels. (Olsen, 2017, para. 4)

Lowers Risk of Cancer

If the cure for cancer were ever found, avocados would definitely play an essential part in the process. This is because research findings have proven that the phytochemical found in avocado can selectively inhibit the growth of precancerous and cancerous cells. It even causes cancer cells' death while simultaneously boosting the proliferation of immune system cells called lymphocytes.

For cancer patients who go through chemotherapy, these phytochemicals have also been shown to decrease chromosomal damage caused by one particular chemotherapy drug, called cyclophosphamide, on the human immune cells.

Apart from these powerful phytochemicals, avocado also contains folate, a nutrient that has shown great potential in protecting against colon, stomach, pancreatic, and cervical cancers. Though it has not yet been verified just how exactly folate reduces cancer risk factors, some researchers believe that it protects against undesirable mutations in DNA and RNA during cell division.

Helps you Lose Weight

We can all see that avocados' calorie content is greater than other fruits and vegetables from its nutritional breakdown. Obviously, most of these calories come from fat, but you don't have to worry since they are healthy and beneficial fats. Several reliable and verified studies have shown that avocados' fat and fiber content help keep you full and satiated.

So, when you consume fat and fiber, your brain receives a signal to turn off your appetite. This, in turn, eliminates any urge to snack throughout the day. If you're still struggling with this habit or want to lose weight easily, avocado is another superfood you should consider adding to your diet!

Provides Anti-aging and Beauty Benefits

Avocado is a popular ingredient in many moisturizing products, including body creams and face masks. This is because it is an excellent source of vitamins E and C, both of which play a great role in promoting your skin's health and vitality.

This powerful combination helps boost collagen production, further reducing signs of aging. The presence of vitamin C may also help speed skin repair and improve chronic skin conditions like eczema and acne. It also prevents your skin from drying out or breaking out. Overall, you get to brag about a healthy and good-looking complexion with the nutrients from avocados.

Promotes a Healthy Pregnancy

Pregnant women need at least 400 micrograms of folate a day to help prevent congenital abnormalities in their babies' brains and spine. Luckily for them, consuming just one avocado offers around 41% of that required amount. Adequate intake of folate also reduces the risk of miscarriage and neural tube defects.

Helps in Preventing and Treating Arthritis and Osteoporosis Symptoms

Avocados contain substances called saponins, which are associated with relief of symptoms in knee osteoarthritis. In addition to this substance, avocado also has a rich amount of Vitamin K, which helps ward off osteoporosis by boosting your bone health and slowing down bone loss. Consuming the required amount of Vitamin K also increases calcium absorption and reduces urinary excretion of calcium.

Often, most people don't know just how important vitamin K is to boost their bone health because of the overpopulation of nutrients like calcium and vitamin D. One avocado can offer you about 26% of the daily value required for Vitamin K.

Helps Promote Eye Health

Avocados contain lutein and zeaxanthin, two phytochemicals that are extremely good for your eyes. These antioxidants protect the tissues in your eyes and help minimize damage from ultraviolet light. It also helps prevent cataracts and macular degeneration.

Improves Digestion

One interesting quality of avocado is that even with its creamy texture, the fruit is actually high in fiber, with approximately 7 grams per half fruit. They're particularly high in insoluble fiber, which is the kind that helps move waste through your body. Its natural fiber content helps prevent constipation, lower colon cancer risk, and maintain a healthy digestive tract.

Lowers Risks of Depression

The benefits of this superfood are not limited to just your physical health; it also stabilizes and improves your mental health. Avocado contains a rich amount of folate, which in this case, helps block the buildup of a substance called homocysteine in your blood. This buildup slows down the circulation and delivery of nutrients to the brain. This can eventually ramp up depression.

Hence, by preventing excess homocysteine build-up, the high folate levels in avocados may help keep depression symptoms at bay. It can also boost the production of serotonin, dopamine, and norepinephrine, the hormones that regulate mood, sleep, and appetite.

How to Include Avocados in Your Meals

We all know that we can easily detect if an avocado is ripe by gently pressing it into the skin. Now in case, you have no choice but to get avocado with firm skin that does not budge, you will have to let it ripen for about 4-5 days before consuming it. However, you can speed up the ripening process by placing the avocado in a paper bag with a banana or apple.

Another problem most people tend to have with avocado is its nutrients oxidizing and turning brown soon after fleshing it, but not to worry! There is a solution. By simply adding lemon juice, you can slow down this process.

Now to the main focus for this section! Avocados have no culinary boundaries thanks to their creamy, rich, fatty texture that blends well with other ingredients! So, here are some ways to add this superfood to your foods and drinks.

1. Cut your avocados into chunks and drizzle them with a bit of olive oil, balsamic vinegar, pepper, and salt. You can also try seasoning it with paprika, cayenne pepper, or lemon juice.

2. Make guacamole, the famous Mexican dish, using only avocados, herbs, and seasonings. Add other great ingredients like corn, pineapple, broccoli, and quinoa when you want to take the dish to the next level!

3. For a healthy breakfast, spread avocado on toast and sandwiches instead of butter or margarine.

4. Give a twist to your regular morning dish of scrambled eggs by adding some sliced avocado when cooked halfway.

5. Use avocado instead of mayonnaise in chicken or egg salad or as a spread on a sandwich.

6. Use it as the base ingredient for your avocado soup or add it to other nutritious soups.

7. Grill your avocados to make a great side dish for your barbecued meat. All you have to do is drizzle lemon juice and brush the sliced halves with olive oil.

8. Prepare smoothies with avocados, green leafy vegetables like Kale, and other fruits.

9. Make avocado ice cream by combining avocado, lime juice, milk, cream, and sugar.

10. Avocados can also be used to make incredible cocktails like margaritas, daiquiris, or martinis.

11. Use them for making bread, desserts, and pancakes.

12. If you have a latex allergy, ensure that you talk to your doctor before adding avocado to your diet. Some people with a severe allergy to latex tend to have symptoms after eating an avocado.

11

KOMBUCHA AND KIMCHI

Have you ever heard of probiotics- the good or friendly kind of microorganisms? Well, whether you have or haven't, we will be exploring two of the most nutritious fermented foods you will ever find! And here, you will learn more about what probiotics are and just how beneficial they are when administered in adequate amounts.

Let's start with Kombucha! For the first time in this book, we are dealing with a drink as a superfood! Sounds contrasting, right? Well, you will see just how much of a nutritious gem it is as you read on. Here is a quick, interesting fact about kombucha; it was discovered as a happy accident about 2,000 years ago. Historical reports claim that a strong cup of sweetened tea was left forgotten, and upon finding it several weeks later, a culture had formed on the top, and the tea beneath was delicious and effervescent.

The making of this fermented drink is just as magical as that story sounds. To get kombucha, you have to make an ordinary brew, usually a mixture of black or green tea and sugar. Then a magic ingredient that transforms ordinary medicine into kombucha is introduced, and it is called S.C.O.B.Y. This is an acronym for symbiotic culture of bacteria and yeast. So, you simply add strains of bacteria and yeast to your sweetened black or green tea, then allow it to ferment to get a tangy kombucha drink!

All of these mixtures usually give the drink a yellow-orange color. Now, during the fermentation process, the yeast in the SCOBY breaks down the sugar in the tea and releases friendly bacteria, which makes Kombucha a rich source of probiotics. In terms of flavor, the drink boasts of a mildly fizzed and slightly sour taste. The distinctive taste comes from acetic acid, which results from the conversion of the sugar ingredient by bacteria and yeasts. Kombucha offers a wide range of medicinal benefits due to the highly effective ingredients used in its production.

Our second fermented superfood is the national food of South Korea! Kimchi is a traditional spicy pickled vegetable dish with a rich history in South Korea dating back over two thousand years. It is traditionally made with fermented vegetables, including cabbage, scallions, and radishes. Consuming the right quantity of this crunchy and flavorful superfood is an easy, low-calorie way to up your vegetable intake. Even beyond all of those, Kimchi also embodies a wide variety of vitamins, minerals, and antioxidants, all of which provide impressive health benefits. One of its main ingredients, Chinese cabbage, boasts of vitamins A and C, at least ten different minerals, and over 34 amino acids.

So, if you are a fan of either tea or spicy food but have never tasted Kombucha and Kimchi, you should certainly give it a try.

Nutritional Breakdown of Kombucha and Kimchi

The nutrients in kombucha can vary depending on the brand and the fermentation process. Some varieties of Kombucha may contain fruit or milk; those will definitely contain more calories. But here are the USDA nutritional stats for 8 ounces of unflavored kombucha:

Calories	30
Fat	0–1 gram
Sodium	2–10 mg
Carbohydrates (in the form of sugar)	4-6 g

Kimchi

According to the USDA, 1-cup (150-gram) serving of commercially prepared kimchi contains the following nutrients:

Calories	23	Vitamin C	22% of the DV
Carbs	4 grams	Vitamin K	55% of the DV
Protein	2 grams	Folate	20% of the DV
Fat	less than 1 gram	Iron	21% of the DV
Fiber	2 grams	Niacin	10% of the DV
Sodium	747 mg	Riboflavin	24% of the DV
Vitamin B6	19% of the Daily Value (DV)		

We must understand that the nutrients in Kimchi vary depending

on the ingredients used and the different ways it is cooked.
Health Benefits of Kombucha and Kimchi

Improves Digestive Health

As we stated in the overview, kombucha and kimchi are fermented superfoods, making them excellent probiotics. In simpler terms, this means that both of them contain a significant amount of the so-called "good bacteria," which, according to several studies, can help you maintain healthy digestion.

Due to their rich probiotics content, both the beverage and food help the body break down food to streamline and improve digestion. They also serve as natural diuretics that help flush waste and toxins more quickly from the body, leaving zero chances for bacterial and fungal infections. A study published in the Journal of Medicinal Food points to kombucha and kimchi's antioxidant activity as the agent for protective digestive health benefits.

Nevertheless, by doing these functions mentioned above effectively, the two superfoods also reduce the negative symptoms of many gastrointestinal disorders, such as inflammatory bowel disease, Irritable Bowel Syndrome, and colon inflammation. Lactobacillus Plantarum — a specific strain common in these probiotic-rich superfoods plays a significant role in this particular aspect. It is also said to help stabilize the digestive tract.

Though more research is needed for this, two compounds, catechins, and isorhamnetin which are also contained in Kombucha, have been shown to possess antiviral properties that could combat some of the organisms that cause gastroenteritis.

Strengthen your Immune System

Those benefits that the probiotic bacteria contained in Kimchi and Kombucha offer in the digestive tract are also carried over to your immune system! This is because the majority of the body's immune functions take place in the gut. Thus, when your gut is in good shape, your immune system is better able to function optimally!

In addition to this, kombucha and kimchi are packed with antioxidants and vitamins B and C, which boost the body's immune system. Particularly, they are very effective in fighting off infections like the common cold and flu.

Support Heart Health

The probiotics in both Kombucha and Kimchi have also shown to be effective in improving our heart health. They positively influence the cholesterol levels by lowering the LDL cholesterol and increasing the good cholesterol levels. Having read the previous chapters, we would be familiar with the fact that lowering elevated low-density lipoprotein cholesterol levels can automatically reduce cardiovascular disease risk, including hypertension and atherosclerosis.

Before we go on to our next point, you must understand that researchers are not sure of the exact ingredients responsible for Kombucha and Kimchi's function. Also, the studies that were able to verify these functions were only done on rats. Nonetheless, the studies hold promising results for humans.

Protects Against Cancer

Most types of cancer are usually characterized by cell mutation and uncontrolled cell growth. However, studies have found that the high concentration of tea polyphenols and antioxidants in kombucha effectively prevents the growth and spread of cancerous cells. The mechanisms involved in the anti-cancer properties of the tea polyphenols are not fully understood. However, some researchers believe that polyphenols block gene mutation and cancer cells' growth while promoting cancer cell death. Other compounds in kombucha that are believed to help inhibit cancer growth include gluconic acid, glucuronic acid, lactic acid, and vitamin C.

Helps Manage Type-2 Diabetes

Many animal studies with promising evidence have confirmed that drinking kombucha may help ease diabetes symptoms in certain diabetic patients. A study published in BMC Complementary and Alternative Medicine discovered that kombucha was even more effective than black tea in reducing the blood glucose levels in diabetic rats.

According to the study, these promising results were due to the fermented tea's ability to slow down the digestion of carbs and inhibit the a-amylase and lipase activity which is usually responsible for higher postprandial (after meal) glucose levels in the pancreas. Kombucha is also said to inhibit the absorption of bad cholesterol and triglycerides (Leech, 2018, para. 13).

May Reduce Inflammation

As previously mentioned, chronic inflammation is linked to just about every health condition, including heart disease, diabetes, arthritis, and respiratory illnesses. Kombucha and Kimchi are two fermented foods that may help reduce it.

In a 2015 study, scientists isolated HDMPPA, one of the principal compounds in kimchi, to experiment with inflammatory proteins' interaction. They discovered that the compound displayed anti-inflammatory properties by blocking and suppressing the release of inflammatory compounds. This, in turn, improved blood vessel health by quelling inflammation. Though further studies are needed, this study shows the promising benefits that consuming Kimchi can provide when reducing inflammatory proteins.

Of course, Kombucha is not left out on this advantage! Kombucha, especially those made from green tea, contains a set of powerful antioxidants called polyphenols. These antioxidants can lessen inflammation in the body, particularly in the intestinal tract.

Prevent Yeast Infections

Vaginal yeast infections usually occur when the Candida fungus, which is normally harmless, multiplies rapidly inside the vagina. Though it can be easily treated, research has discovered that this fungus may sometimes develop antibiotic resistance, which calls for the search for natural treatments. Now here is where Kombucha and Kimchi come in as superheroes to save the day!

Their rich probiotics and healthy bacteria, especially certain Lactobacillus strains, may help fight Candida and prevent yeast infections. One test-tube study even found that multiple strains isolated from kimchi displayed antimicrobial activity against this fungus.

Nevertheless, kombucha seems to be more effective in this case. This is because, along with its probiotics, it also contains acetic acid, which is one of the main substances produced during its fermentation. Studies have shown that acetic acid has strong antibacterial properties, capable of killing many potentially harmful microorganisms, including the Candida yeasts.

Interestingly, these antimicrobial effects suppress the growth of only undesirable bacteria and yeasts, and they do not affect the beneficial, probiotic bacteria and yeasts involved in the kombucha fermentation.

Improves the Health of Your Liver

Kombucha may play a significant role in improving liver health and reducing liver inflammation due to its potential ability to detoxify the body. If you consume the drink regularly, its antioxidant-rich nature may reduce how hard your liver has to work. Some research, including a Pharmaceutical Biology study from 2014, suggests that consuming kombucha may help protect against drug-induced liver damages. This was concluded after the rats that were administered kombucha showed decreased thiobarbituric acid reactive substances in their livers.

How to Include Kombucha and Kimchi in Your Meals

Kombucha

Now that we have confirmed that kombucha is a probiotic-rich tea with many potential health benefits, it's the perfect time to take advantage of the multi-beneficial tea.

You can purchase it in stores or make it yourself at home. However, if you are making kombucha at home, you must be extremely careful as it can ferment for too long. It is also very easy for the drink to become contaminated, especially when you are not making it in a sterile environment. And we don't mean to scare you, but over fermentation or contamination can cause adverse health problems like food poisoning.

For this reason, it is a much safer option to buy a bottled kombucha at reliable health-food stores, grocery stores, or even online. Actually, commercial kombuchas happen to be tastier. You'll find them in a variety of flavors that will surely tempt your taste buds.

They also usually contain less than 0.5% alcohol until the homemade kombucha, which may have up to 3% alcohol. Nevertheless, ensure that you check the ingredients and, by all means, avoid brands that are high in added sugar.

Now we know you might be thinking, " why so many precautions?" Well, it is for your good, and you will indeed thank us later for this! If you adhere to all these precautions, then kombucha can be a pretty exciting ingredient for you to experiment with your culinary creativity in the kitchen. Beyond consuming it as a refreshing beverage, here are some ideas you can try to include Kombucha in your meals;

1. Use kombucha in place of vinegar for your salad dressing and condiments such as ketchup and mustard.

2. Soak your grains overnight in kombucha tea; after mixing it with water and then drain the water and use the grains for baking for healthier, fluffier, and tastier bread, cakes, and muffins. Kombucha actually helps break down the complex elements of grains.

3. Need an acidic ingredient for any of your cocktail recipes? Use kombucha in place of sweet and sour mix or as a healthy alternative to sodas.

4. You can also take advantage of the acidity of a long-brewed kombucha drink by using it to marinate any meat, be it pork,

chicken, beef, even lamb, shrimp, or fish.

5. Kombucha can be blended with fruit or juice to add to a frizzing sour flavor.

6. It can also be frozen to make popsicles or granitas.

7. Give your hearty winter soup the perfect finishing and the perfect balancing sour note that only a little kombucha can offer.

Kimchi

Just like Kombucha, buying kimchi in health-stores, grocery stores, or online is a much safer option to avoid cases of over fermentation and contamination. Here are some creative ways in which you can incorporate kimchi into your diet.

1. You can enjoy your kimchi straight out of the jar for a bit of snack at any time of the day.

2. Stir some finely chopped kimchi into your steamed or fried rice to give it a nice little kick of tangy spice. In the case of fried rice, make sure to stir the kimchi right at the last minute after everything is fried.

3. Add kimchi into any kind of cake or savory pancake to give it a nice bit of crunchy texture and spicy-tart flavor.

4. Adding kimchi to a tomato base for a braise lends an unexpected twist to a classic preparation.

5. Kimchi is that medicinal spice that makes a great addition to the traditional Korean tofu stew when it comes to helping you battle any cold or flu that comes your way.

6. You can ditch tomatoes and use butter and kimchi to make pasta sauce.

12

OLIVE OIL

It has been quite a long journey, and we finally made it to the last superfood we will discuss! But it isn't over just yet. Now, no one can deny that olive oil is a special kitchen ingredient! The culinary experts and creatives among us will surely agree that the world-renowned chefs have recommended this gem for cooking way too many times! Now let me properly introduce you to the wonderful world of olive oil.

First of all, you should know that olive oil is the natural oil extracted from olives, the fruit of the olive tree. It has been a major component of the Mediterranean cultures for thousands of years, dating back to the Ancient Greeks and Romans. Guess what? Olive oil was popularly called 'Liquid Gold' in those days. Even to date, it remains the most popular cooking oil in the region. You might be curious as to why these people are so obsessed with olive oil. Researchers have discovered that people from the Mediterranean, where olive oil is grown and consumed the most, have the lowest mortality rates globally when it comes to many chronic diseases. We don't know about you, but this is more than enough reason to get obsessed with olive oil.

Nowadays, there are three main grades of olive oil, namely refined, virgin, and extra virgin. Of these three varieties, extra virgin olive oil is the least processed and healthiest type of olive oil. As such, it is your best option if you truly want to get all the health benefits we will be discussing very soon.

Compared to every other cooking oil, olive oil is the most uniquely blessed oil with the powerful potential to deliver impressive health benefits from improved cholesterol levels and better mood to stronger bones and the treatment of chronic and degenerative diseases. It results from highly effective fatty acids, bioactive compounds, antioxidants, and other nutrients in the oil. Let's see what its nutritional profile entails.

Nutritional Breakdown of Olive Oil

According to the USDA, one tablespoon of olive oil (14g) contains the following nutritional profile:

Calories	120
Total Fat	14 grams
Saturated Fat	2.2 grams
Polyunsaturated Fat	1.8 grams
Monounsaturated Fat	10 grams
Vitamin E	13% of the Daily Value (DV)
Vitamin K	7% of the DV

This particular amount of olive oil does not provide any percentage of cholesterol, sodium, and potassium.

Health Benefits of Olive Oil

Strongly Promotes Cardiovascular health

Olive oil has long been popularized as a heart-healthy fat, and this is because of many reasons. Several studies have shown that people who consume the Mediterranean diet, which has olive oil as its main source of fat, appear to have a higher life expectancy, including a lower chance of dying from cardiovascular diseases, than people who follow other diets. These researchers believe that olive oil contributes largely to this impressive record.

But how exactly does olive oil achieve this particular health benefit? Some studies revealed that oleic acid, a type of monounsaturated fat found in high quantities in olive oil, helps reduce the risk of heart disease when used in place of other fat sources. However, another study suggested that the polyphenols in extra virgin olive oil are responsible for protecting cardiovascular disease.

Despite their conflicting knowledge requiring the exact mechanism responsible for olive oil's heart-protecting functions, some experts have termed it "The standard in preventive medicine." In fact, the Food and Drug Administration (FDA) has claimed that replacing fats and oils higher in saturated fat with 1.5 tablespoons (22 ml) of extra virgin olive oil each day will reduce the risk of cardiovascular disease and inflammation. Thus, at this point, we can safely conclude that olive oil is indeed a superfood that those who have heart disease or are at a high risk of developing it must consider incorporating into their diets.

Helps Prevent Breast Cancer

Women in Mediterranean countries where olive oil is a staple food tend to have a lower risk of breast cancers. Many researchers believe that their regular consumption of olive oil may also be responsible for this. A study conducted in Saudi Arabia found that oleuropein, a natural compound found in olive leaf, has potential anti-breast cancer properties.

Apart from this, the antioxidants in olive oil have also proven to reduce oxidative damage caused by free radicals, which is believed to be a leading driver of cancer. So that you know, the effectiveness of olive oil is not restricted to just breast cancer. However, the results for the other types of cancer aren't as promising as this one.

Prevents Alzheimer's Disease

By now, we should all be familiar with the fact that Alzheimer's disease is one of the most common neurodegenerative diseases highly affected by oxidative stress. However, the good news is that the polyphenols in extra virgin olive oil, particularly oleocanthal, can function as potent antioxidants that may help counter oxidative stress. According to Scientific American, oleocanthal in olive oil can help prevent Alzheimer's disease. This claim was given more credibility by a 2019 American study on mice where oleocanthal-rich olive oil was discovered to help restore healthy blood-brain barrier function and reduce neuroinflammation in a way that may slow the progression of Alzheimer's. Though more research is needed in this area, other studies support the possibility of olive oil having the same kind of improvement in humans who have Alzheimer's.

Strengthens Bones

There is about a 50% chance that the first thing that came to your mind when you saw this point was calcium! True or false? If our assumption is, in fact, true, then you should understand that calcium isn't the only nutrient that makes your bones strong.

In a study that involves men consuming a Mediterranean diet, it was discovered that olive oil might be very effective in promoting strong bones. Here is how it happens; inflammation in the body tends to actually turn on the osteoclast cells, which are well-known for breaking down bone. However, researchers believe that anti-inflammatory polyphenols in olive oil trigger mechanisms that help prevent bone breakdown and stimulate bone formation. Also, the consumption of olive oil may result in higher levels of osteocalcin, indicating healthy bone formation in the body.

Reduces Risk of Stroke

Second only to heart disease, stroke is the world's leading cause of death. It is usually caused by a disturbance of blood flow to the brain, either due to a blood clot or bleeding. Studies have shown that the daily consumption of olive oil, especially the extra virgin variety, can help prevent strokes in the elderly. This isn't just a mere claim! The relationship between olive oil and stroke risk has been studied extensively. In fact, a large review of studies conducted in 841,000 people found that olive oil was the only source of monounsaturated fat associated with a reduced risk of stroke.

How does it happen? Olive oil contains minimum levels of saturated and polyunsaturated fats and the highest level of monounsaturated fat – around 75 to 80%. This property gives the oil the ability to control blood cholesterol levels, building good cholesterol and HDL in the body. Olive oil can also help prevent unwanted blood clotting, which is a major risk factor for stroke.

Serves as Remedy for Constipation

Olive oil is rich in monounsaturated fats, vitamins E and K, iron, omega-3 and 6 fatty acids, and other antioxidants. These nutrients basically help in improving your overall health, including the digestion, by consuming olive oil, whether by drinking it directly or using it as an ingredient. Researchers have verified that it offers very effective results in completely preventing constipation. In addition to its nutrients, the texture of olive oil also stimulates your digestive system, making the food particles move smoothly through the gastrointestinal tract and colon. By increasing the food's mobility through your colon without any problem, the oil also helps speed up bowel evacuation and eventually eliminates any constipation risk. In cases of infections, olive oil contains a set of antioxidants called polyphenols which may reduce inflammation of the GI tract and foster the growth of healthy bifidobacterial in your gut.

Improves Nail Health

Many people don't know that their nails often say a lot about their state of health. Why else do you think your doctor sometimes checks your nails when you feel sick or look pale? However, we must also emphasize that having dull, lifeless, brittle nails doesn't necessarily have to be because of certain ailments or a poor state of health; it could be due to a lack of care on your part. Luckily, by consuming olive oil, we can solve these problems, as it is a natural and easy way to improve nail health. Always remember that it is only when your nails are looking healthy that you can freely use and flaunt that trendy nail art for your next big birthday party or hangout!

Promotes Skin Health

The benefits of olive oil are not limited to just improving your physical health. It is also beneficial for enhancing beauty in both males and females. This oil contains a good amount of vitamin E, an antioxidant that protects the skin from various external factors, especially the harsh sun rays, which can cause serious ailments like psoriasis and skin cancer. Olive oil can also help in the treatment of skin inflammation and acne.

Some people even take advantage of its texture and make the oil their go-to non-sticky moisturizer. One fantastic feature that beauticians have discovered about the oil is that it suits all skin types and stays fresh for a long period of time. In case you are worried about your skin sagging and developing wrinkles due to aging, then you might want to try adding olive oil to your diet or even applying directly to your skin to delay those signs of aging.

How to Include Olive Oil in Your Meals

Before we even explore how you can add olive oil to your meals, you must understand that purchasing the right kind of olive oil is extremely important. Choosing extra virgin olive oil or maybe the multipurpose fine virgin oil is your healthiest option. These varieties of olive oil undergo less processing and are more likely to retain their antioxidants and bioactive compound contents than those refined ones. They are also suitable for cooking and drinking directly.

Be aware that you must also be very careful as there are so many types of fake extra virgin oil. Nowadays, many oils labeled "extra virgin" have actually been diluted with other refined oils. Hence, you must always examine the labels carefully to ensure you're getting the real extra virgin olive oil. Taking your time to read the ingredients list and check for quality certification can save you from many health problems in the end. Now in terms of storage, make sure that you use up the content of an open bottle of olive oil within 3-6 months or less.

Not only does olive oil enhance savory and sweet dishes, but it also enables us to satisfy our appetite and enjoy the upgraded pleasing tastes in our mouths without feeling any ounces of guilt since we know it is an embodiment of wonderful health-boosting properties. Want to know what that feels like? Here are some ways you can include the superfood in your meals.

1. Drizzle the oil straight onto the salad or add it to a salad dressing.
2. Use in marinades for meat, fish, poultry, and vegetables.
3. Substitute butter with olive oil when baking especially savory loaves of bread and sweets such as cakes, cookies, and other desserts.
4. Instead of butter or margarine, you can also use olive oil as a healthy dip for your bread.
5. You can also make a tasty, heart-healthy dip by mixing olive oil with cooked white beans and garlic in a food processor, then seasoning the mixture to taste with your favorite herbs.
6. Use it instead of other fats when frying or sautéing.
7. To seal in the meaty flavor and create a crispy exterior for your grilled meat, brush olive oil on it before cooking.
8. Use olive oil when making your sauces.
9. Sprinkle on brown rice.
10. Drizzle a little over your cooked pasta or vegetables to give it

a burst of flavor.

While trying out all of these creative culinary styles, please note that olive oil has a higher smoke point than most other oils, usually about 400 degrees Fahrenheit.

13

15 RECIPES TO IMPROVE HEALTH USING THE SUPERFOODS

At this point, you surely will not have any more doubt as to how beneficial the so-called "superfoods" are. Together, we have deeply and thoroughly explored the nutritious and medicinal powers of over 20 superfoods. Still, we cannot afford to leave it since the major aim is to equip you with the best tool kit that will ensure you really get started on this journey.

Although these foods are called "superfoods," that doesn't imply they will be super complicated to prepare. For this section, we have put together a list of very simple, healthy recipes that will be of great help to everyone from the culinary experts who want to explore their creativity in the kitchen to those of us that are inexperienced in the kitchen or may sometimes not be in the mood to cook an elaborate meal. Each of these featured recipes includes at least one superfood discussed in the book. So, get your cooking utensils and ingredients ready because these recipes are guaranteed to produce a nutrient-packed meal!

STUFFED BELL PEPPERS

Prep Time: 20 minutes
Cook Time: 1 hour
Total Time: 1 hour 20 minutes

Ingredients

6 bell peppers any color, or a combination of colors
2 teaspoons olive oil
1 1/2 pounds ground beef
1/2 cup onion, finely chopped
2 teaspoons garlic, minced
1 1/2 cups cooked white rice
Salt and pepper to taste
15 ounce can tomato sauce
1/2 teaspoon Italian seasoning
1 1/2 cups mozzarella cheese shredded, divided use
2 tablespoons parsley, chopped
Cooking spray

Directions

1. Start by preheating your oven to 350 degrees F. Then coat a large baking dish with cooking spray.
2. Slice the tops off the 6 bell peppers; remove the ribs and seeds inside.
3. Place the side of the peppers down in the baking dish. Add 1 1/2 cups of water to the dish and then cover it with foil and bake for 25 minutes.
4. As you wait for the peppers to cook, prepare the filling. Start by heating the olive oil in a large pan over medium heat.
5. Add the ground beef and season it with salt and pepper. Cook this for 5-6 minutes, breaking up the meat with a spatula, until it is cooked. Add the onion to the pan and cook for 3-4

minutes or until softened. Then add the garlic and cook for another 30 seconds.

6. Now combine the rice, tomato sauce, and Italian seasoning. Stir in 1/2 cup of cheese as well as salt and pepper to taste.

7. Remove the peppers from the oven and drain off the water. Turn the peppers over and fill each one with the beef mixture.

8. Again, top each pepper with the remaining cheese—cover1-inch and bake for 20 minutes. Uncover and bake for another 10 minutes or until cheese is melted and browned and peppers are tender.

9. Sprinkle the stuffed bell peppers with parsley, and then serve.

Credit: IPR Fresh

HEALTHY ORANGE CHICKEN

Prep Time: 10 minutes
Cook Time: 35 minutes
Total Time: 45 minutes
Yields: 4 servings.

Ingredients

2 lbs. boneless, skinless chicken breasts
4 cups steamed broccoli or green beans
2 tablespoons toasted sesame oil

For the sauce

2 cups orange juice
1/4 cup chicken broth (optional but with no salt added)
1/4 cup coconut amino
3 tablespoons honey
1 teaspoon garlic powder
2 teaspoons fresh ginger
1/2 tablespoon orange zest
1/2 teaspoon pepper

Directions

1. Clean and cut chicken into 1-inch cubes.
2. Heat the sesame oil in a large frying pan. Cook the chicken until the edges are brown and slightly crispy. That should be taking approximately 12-15 minutes.
3. As the chicken is cooking, stir together the orange juice, chicken broth, coconut amino, honey, garlic powder, fresh ginger, orange zest, and pepper in a separate bowl.
4. Once the chicken is thoroughly cooked, remove it from the pan and place it off to the side in a separate bowl.
5. Now pour the sauce mixture into the same pan you used in cooking the chicken.

6. Bring the sauce mixture to a boil for about 15-20 minutes, stirring every minute or so until it starts to thicken. Once you scrape the pan and pull away from the pan, you will know that the sauce has thickened. Note that sauce should be bubbling the entire time.

7. At that point, add the cooked chicken back in and stir to coat it with the sauce.

8. Serve over steamed broccoli or green beans or rice/quinoa.

9. Sprinkle with sesame seeds and enjoy!

LOW-CARB WATERMELON SMOOTHIE

Prep Time: 5 mins
Total Time: 5 mins
Yields: 4 cups

Ingredients

2 cups watermelon (cubed and chilled)
Juice of 1 lime
5 drops stevia liquid (or to taste)
5-10 fresh mint leaves (to taste)
3 cups of ice
½ cup soy milk

Directions

1. Add the watermelon cubes, lime juice, stevia, soy milk, and mint into a blender.
2. Blend until the mixture is completely smooth.
3. Add the ice and pulse until the smoothie is incorporated. Serve immediately

BLUEBERRY OATMEAL MUFFINS

Prep Time: 40 minutes
Cook Time: 20 minutes
Total Time: 1 hour, 10 minutes
Yield: 12 muffins

Ingredients
1 cup (240ml) milk
1 cup (80g) old-fashioned whole rolled oats
1 and 1/4 cups (156g) all-purpose flour (spoon & leveled)
1 teaspoon baking powder
1/2 teaspoon baking soda
1/2 teaspoon ground cinnamon
1/2 teaspoon salt
1/2 cup (115g) unsalted butter, melted and slightly cooled
1/2 cup (120ml) honey
1 large egg
1 teaspoon pure vanilla extract
1 cup (190g) fresh or frozen blueberries (see note if using frozen)

Directions
1. Combine your milk and oats in a bowl and set aside for 20 minutes,1-inchof so the oats and get puffed up and soaked up with some moisture. If you find the oats haven't soaked up any moisture after 20 minutes, stir it and wait for another 10 minutes.
2. Preheat your oven to 425°F (218°C). Spray a 12-count muffin pan with nonstick spray or use cupcake liners.
3. Mix your dry ingredients; flour, baking powder, baking soda, cinnamon, and salt, and then mix them in a large bowl until combined. Set aside.
4. In another medium bowl, whisk the melted butter, honey, egg, and vanilla extract until combined.

5. Now pour the wet ingredients into the dry ingredients, and stir a few times.
6. Add the blueberries and soaked oats without draining the milk. Gently fold everything together just until combined. Spoon the batter into liners, filling them all the way to the top.
7. Top with oats and a light sprinkle of coconut sugar, if desired.
8. Bake for 5 minutes at 425. While still keeping the muffins in the oven, reduce the oven temperature to 350°F (177°C). Bake for an additional 16-17 minutes or until a toothpick inserted in the center comes out clean.
9. Usually, it takes a total time of 22-22 minutes to bake these muffins in the oven but for mini muffins, bake 11-13 minutes at 350°F (177°C).)
10. Allow the muffins to cool for 5 minutes in the muffin pan, and then transfer to a wire rack to continue cooling.
11. Blueberry muffins stay fresh covered at room temperature for a few days, then transfer to the fridge for up to 1 week.

Credit: Bloomingfoods

ROASTED PUMPKIN SEEDS

Prep Time: 10 mins
Cook Time: 15 mins
Total Time: 25 mins
Yields: 12 servings

Ingredients
¾ cup raw pumpkin seeds
1 tablespoon olive oil
½ teaspoon kosher salt
¼ teaspoon garlic powder
¼ teaspoon paprika, (optional)
⅛ teaspoon black pepper

Directions
1. Preheat the oven to 350°F (177°C).
2. Wash the pumpkin seeds in a colander to remove the pulp and fibers. Dry it thoroughly with a towel.
3. Next, combine pumpkin seeds, olive oil, salt, garlic powder, paprika (if desired), and black pepper.
4. Lightly grease a sheet pan with a good amount of olive oil and then spread the seasoned pumpkin seeds on the sheet pan.
5. Bake for about 12 to 15 minutes until the seeds are toasted and crunchy. Make sure to stir every 5 minutes while it is toasting, and check for crunchiness with each stir by tasting a seed.
6. Transfer the roasted pumpkin seeds to a bowl to cool down. Then serve.

HEIRLOOM CARROT PASTA WITH A SUNFLOWER CHEESE SAUCE

Ingredients

1/4 cup sunflower seeds

1/2 cup water

1 tablespoon soy sauce (tamari for gluten-free)

1/2 teaspoon smoked paprika

1 yellow onion

2 cloves of garlic

1 teaspoon gluten-free white miso

1 tablespoon nutritional yeast

Directions

1. Dissolve the sea salt in the 1/2 cup of water. Pour in the sunflower seeds, then cover the bowl with breathable material, leave to soak overnight or for at least 8 hours.
2. Heat the olive oil and sauté 1 chopped yellow onion and 2 garlic cloves in a pan. Cook until the onion is translucent.
3. Drain the water from the soaked sunflower seeds and rinse them with clean water. Puree the seeds in a blender with the cooked garlic and onion.
4. Add the soy sauce, smoked paprika, white miso, nutritional yeast, and another 1/2 cup of water. Then blend all until smooth.
5. The heirloom carrot pasta cut the 4 large heirloom carrots into thin strips, using a julienne peeler or spiralizer to make the task easier for you. Your goal should be to make pasta-like strips.

6. Pour a bit of water into a pot, bring to a boil. Put the pasta-like carrot strips into a steamer basket and place the basket in the pot. Cover and steam the carrots for a minute.

7. Serve the carrot pasta in 2 bowls, pour sauce on top, and serve with some fresh alfalfa sprouts or a handful of roasted pumpkin seeds.

BROCCOLI AND EGG FRIED RICE

Prep and Cook Time: 20 mins
Yields: 2 servings

Ingredients
Sesame oil.
2 eggs, lightly beaten
2 cloves of fat garlic, finely chopped
200g (7ounces) broccoli, cut into florets
1/2 cup frozen mixed vegetables (peas, sweet corn & carrots), thawed
2 cups cooked rice
2 Tablespoons of light soy sauce
1 Tablespoon of Indonesian sweet soy sauce

Directions
1. Firstly, make your scrambled egg because no fried rice is complete without it. So, heat oil in a pan over medium flame and when the oil is hot, pour the lightly beaten eggs. Cook until the eggs are scrambled.
2. Turn the fire to low, then use a spatula to push the eggs to a side and add garlic. Without mixing the garlic with the egg, sauté it until aromatic and very lightly brown.
3. Add in your broccoli with a pinch of salt, mixing it with the rest of the ingredients in the pan. Cook the broccoli florets over medium heat until they turn bright green, especially the stalk section.
4. Next, add the mixed vegetables and cooked rice. The rice needs to be cold before cooking. Now stir to combine well.
5. Sauté the mixture for about a minute over high heat, then turn the flame to low, add soy sauce and sweet soy sauce. Stir again to combine all ingredients. Turn the flame to high again; cook the fried rice for another 20 seconds. Then Serve immediately.

LEMONY MUSHROOM PASTA

Prep Time: 20 mins
Yields: 4 servings

Ingredients

1 pound portabella mushrooms, full size or baby
8 ounces of pasta
3 tablespoons of olive oil
1 large clove garlic, chopped
1 sprig thyme leaves, stripped from the stalks (optional)
1 dried cayenne pepper pod, deseeded and broken into large pieces (optional)
3 medium shallots, thinly sliced
1 tablespoon Italian parsley, roughly chopped
Juice of 1 lemon
Salt and pepper to taste

Directions

1. Start with your mushrooms and cut the stalks from them. If it has roots, remove them, and cut the remaining stalks into chunks. Use a damp cloth to wipe the caps and cut them into -inch dice.
2. Heat the olive oil over medium-high heat until it starts to ripple. Add in the garlic, thyme, and cayenne pepper. Cook the mixture until the garlic starts to color.
3. Then add the shallots and parsley. Sauté until the shallots start to color.
4. Make sure it is softened before adding the mushrooms. Add a small amount of salt and pepper to taste. Sauté until the mushrooms start to give up their juices and color.
5. When that is fully done, take the pan off the heat and pour the lemon juice over the content.
6. Mix everything well; cover the pan and let it sit while you focus

on cooking the pasta.

7. Cook pasta according to package instructions. When the pasta is done, drain and toss the dripping pasta with the mushrooms.

8. Serve your meal with a grind of black pepper and freshly grated Parmesan cheese, if you desired.

Credit: Cook for Your Life

BASQUE-STYLE SALMON STEW

Prep Time: 10 mins
Cook Time: 25 mins
Yields: 4 servings

Ingredients
1 tbsp olive oil
3 mixed peppers, deseeded and sliced
1 large onion, thinly sliced
400g baby potatoes, unpeeled and halved
2 tsp smoked paprika
2 garlic cloves, sliced
2 tsp dried thyme
400g can of chopped tomatoes
4 salmon fillets
1 tbsp chopped parsley for serving (optional)

Directions
1. Heat the olive oil in a large pan and add the peppers, onion, and potatoes. While stirring regularly, cook for 5-8 mins until golden.
2. Then add the paprika, garlic, thyme, and tomatoes. Bring to them to boil, stir and cover, then turn down the heat and simmer for 12 mins.
3. Add a splash of water if the sauce becomes too thick. Season the stew and lay the salmon on top, skin side down.
4. Place the lid back on and simmer for another 8 mins until the salmon is cooked through.
5. Scatter with parsley, if you desire and serve.

SLOW COOKER TURKEY MEATBALLS

Prep Time: 1 hr.
Cook Time: 5 hrs.
Yields: 4 - 5 servings

Ingredients

1 tbsp rapeseed oil
1 onion, finely chopped
2 carrots, finely diced
2 celery sticks, finely diced
2 garlic cloves, thinly sliced
500g carton tomato passata
2 tbsp chopped parsley
400g lean minced turkey
4 tbsp porridge oats
Pinch of paprika
1 garlic clove, crushed
Spray of oil

Directions

1. If necessary, you can heat the slow cooker first. Heat the oil in a non-stick frying pan, then add the onion, carrots, celery, and garlic and fry gently for a minute.
2. Pour in the passata, add the parsley, and stir, then transfer the lot to the slow cooker.
3. Now let's focus on making the meatballs tip the minced turkey into a large bowl. Add the oats, paprika, garlic, and plenty of black pepper, and mix everything with your hands.
4. Divide the mixture into 20 lumps about a walnut's size and roll each piece into a meatball.

5. Spray or run a non-stick pan with a little oil and gently cook the meatballs until they start to brown.
6. Add them to the tomato base and cook on low for 5 hours.
7. Serve over rice or pasta if you like, or with a green salad.

Credit: Pressure King Pro

ROASTED SWEET POTATOES WITH HONEY AND CINNAMON

Prep Time: 15 min
Cook Time: 30 min
Yields: 4 servings

Ingredients

4 sweet potatoes, peeled and cut into 1-inch cubes
1/3 cup extra-virgin olive oil (you can add a little more for drizzling on the potatoes after roasted)
1/4 cup honey
2 teaspoons ground cinnamon
Salt and freshly ground black pepper

Directions

1. Preheat your oven to 375 degrees F.
2. Get a roasting tray and lay the cube-shaped sweet potatoes out in a single layer. Drizzle the oil, honey, cinnamon, salt, and pepper over the potatoes.
3. Get the tray into the oven and roast for 25 to 30 minutes or until tender.
4. Take the roasted sweet potatoes out of the oven and transfer them to a serving platter.
5. Drizzle with more extra-virgin olive oil if you desire.

SPICY CHICKEN & AVOCADO WRAPS

Prep Time: 5 mins
Cook Time: 8 mins
Yields: 2 Servings

Ingredients
1 chicken breast (117approx. 180g), thinly sliced at an angle
1 avocado, halved and stoned
Squeezed juice of ½ lime
½ tsp mild chili powder
1 garlic clove, chopped
1 tsp olive oil
2 seeded wraps
1 roasted red pepper from a jar, sliced
A few sprigs of coriander, chopped

Directions
1. Put your sliced chicken breast in a bowl and mix it well with lime juice, chili powder, and garlic.
2. Heat the olive oil in a non-stick frying pan, then fry the chicken for a couple of mins. Make sure to keep an eye on it as the chicken will cook very quickly.
3. As you are doing so, warm the wraps following the pack instructions. Or, if you have a gas hob, heat them over the flame to slightly char them. Do not let them dry out, or they will be difficult to roll.
4. Squash half an avocado onto each wrap, add the peppers to the pan to warm them through.
5. Next, pile the chicken mixture onto the wraps and sprinkle it over the coriander.
6. Roll up the wraps; cut in half, and eat with your fingers.
   Credit: Irish Country Magazine & BBC Good Food Middle East

KIMCHI PANCAKES

Prep Time: 5 minutes
Cook Time: 20 minutes
Total Time: 25 minutes
Yields: 4 big servings

Ingredients

2 & 1/2 cup all-purpose flour
2 & 1/2 cup water
1/2 tsp fine sea salt
1 large egg, beaten
2 cups or about 420g Kimchi
1 Tbsp Kimchi liquid
5 or about 100g ice cubes
2 green chilies (optional)
1 red chili (optional)
Some vegetable cooking oil, preferably rice bran oil
Homemade Kimchi pancake dipping sauce to serve

Directions

1. To make the batter, start by sieving the flour and the salt. Add the water and whisk it well.
2. Add the beaten egg, kimchi, kimchi liquid, and chilies. Mix them well. Add the ice cubes to keep the batter cold.
3. Now preheat a pan or skillet until well heated. Spread a generous amount of cooking oil all over the pan.
4. Pour the batter and cook it on high heat initially for 10 to 20 seconds, then reduce the heat to medium to low. Make sure this temperature setting remains the same till you finish.
5. As it cooks, press the pancake with the spatula a couple of times to make it crispy.
6. Then turn the pancake over when the bottom is cooked, and the top is also partially cooked. This will make it easy to turn

the pancake.

7. When both sides are cooked, slice it into easy-to-bite-size pieces. Then serve with some Korean pancake dipping sauce if you desire.

Credit: Brighton and Hove Food Partnership

APPLE-GINGER KOMBUCHA

Active Time: 10 Mins
Total Time: 240 Hours
Yields: 6 servings (serving size: 16 ounces)

Ingredients
3 1/2 quarts water
1 cup granulated sugar
6 bags black tea
2 bags of green tea
1 cup starter tea (prepared kombucha)
1-gallon jar 5 (16-ounce) glass airtight bottles
1 clean plastic bottle
12 tablespoons apple juice
12 slices fresh, peeled ginger, from 2-inch knob ginger root

Directions
1. Pour water into a large saucepan, add sugar and bring it to a boil.
2. Add the black and green tea bags, and remove them from heat. Let it steep for 15 minutes. Remove tea bags, and let the water cool for about 30 minutes.
3. Pour the cooled tea into a gallon jar. Add starter tea and SCOBY. Cover the gallon jar with paper towels, and seal with a rubber band.
4. Set aside, covered, for 7 days at 70°F, out of direct sunlight.
5. After a week, pour the tea into 5 glass bottles and then into 1 plastic bottle through a funnel. Add the apple juice and add 2 slices of ginger.
6. Seal the bottle and set it aside at room temperature or in the refrigerator for 3-5 days.
7. When a plastic bottle feels tight to the touch, the kombucha is ready to be consumed.

CREAMED ONIONS

Prep Time: 35 mins
Cook Time: 20 mins
Total Time: 55 mins
Yield: 8 servings

Ingredients

2 pounds small white onions
¼ cup butter
¼ cup all-purpose flour
2 cups half-and-half
1 pinch ground nutmeg
1 pinch salt
2 drops hot pepper sauce

Directions

1. Cut off the ends of the onions and place them in a large pot of water. Bring to boil; drain the water and cool slightly.
2. Then slip the skins off and return the onions to water. Simmer until tender.
3. In a saucepan, melt butter and gradually stir in flour. Keep stirring until the mixture is smooth. Cook over low heat for 5 minutes, stirring constantly.
4. In another separate saucepan, scald half and half, gradually whisk into butter mixture. Add nutmeg, salt, and pepper sauce; add onions and cook until thick and smooth.

2 WEEK MEAL PLAN - USING SUPERFOODS

Most of us tend to be very busy because of family, work, schooling, or other activities in our daily lives. Thus, we have little or no time to create a realistic meal plan to incorporate enough of these nutrient-packed superfoods into our diets. With this plan, however, you can easily learn to make simple and delicious meals for yourself and your family. And you know what's even more fantastic about it? You get to experience zero guilt and great assurance, knowing that you are intentionally treating your body with the goodness it deserves.

WEEK 1

	DAY 1	DAY 2	DAY 3	DAY 4	DAY 5	DAY 6	DAY 7
Breakfast	Blueberry oatmeal muffins	Mug scrambled eggs	Roasted sweet potatoes with honey and cinnamon	Stir-fried mustard greens with eggs and garlic	Apple and almond butter toast	Yogurt Granola Parfait	Fried eggs and veggie sandwich served on a sweet potato slice
Morning Snack	¼ cup of roasted pumpkin seeds	Mixed frozen fruits slices – strawberries, watermelons, cherries, or oranges	Celery sticks with 2 tbsp cream cheese	Apple and peanut butter	Kale chips	Cucumber slices with hummus	Turkey roll-ups
Lunch	Kimchi bowl with red curry almond sauce	Open-faced garden tuna sandwich	Lentil soup and salad	Curried Chicken Apple Wraps	Rainbow Buddha with Cashew Tahini Sauce	Ginger roasted salmon and broccoli and ½ cup of cauliflower rice	Round pork served in cabbage
Afternoon Snack	Peanut Butter-oat Energy Balls	Vegan oat chocolate chip cookies	Greek yogurt with berries	Veggie spring rolls	Berries with honey-ginger dip	Peppermint tea and dark chocolate chips	Cottage cheese with flax seeds and cinnamon
Dinner	Salmon with pineapple salsa	Heirloom carrot pasta with sunflower cheese sauce	Greek Mac and Cheese Casseroles with a portion of steamed broccoli	Steamed brown rice with chicken and vegetable stir fry	Slow cooker Turkey Meatballs	Thin-crust veggie pizza	Veggie Korean bibimbap, with apple-ginger Kombucha drink

WEEK 2

	DAY 1	DAY 2	DAY 3	DAY 4	DAY 5	DAY 6	DAY 7
Breakfast	Vegetable omelet (red pepper, spinach, onion, and mushroom)	Apple Cinnamon Quinoa Bowl	Whole grain toast with smashed avocado	Blueberry-Banana Overnight Oats	Sunflower and avocado toast	Kimchi pancakes	Baked eggs in portabella mushrooms
Morning Snack	1 medium orange	Plain Greek yogurt topped with berries and topped with nuts	Low-carb watermelon smoothie	Carrot cake energy bar	Veggie and Hummus Sandwich	½ cup blueberries and 1 cup green tea	Cantaloupe slices wrapped in prosciutto
Lunch	Frittata made with smoked salmon and asparagus	Avocado and shrimp chopped salad	Green Salad with Edamame and Beets	Stuffed mushrooms with meatballs, avocado, tomato, and alfalfa sprouts	Sweet potatoes and black beans chili	Mini burgers made with turkey, bacon, plantains and served with a cilantro aioli sauce	Spicy chicken and avocado wraps
Afternoon Snack	Dried unsweetened coconut	Red bell pepper with guacamole	½ cup of sunflower seeds	Greek yogurt and some berries	Cinnamon flax seed pudding	Beef sticks	Dark chocolate and almonds
Dinner	Broccoli and egg fried rice	Loaded Garden Pizzalad	Lemony mushroom pasta	Turkey Black Beans Burgers and sweet potato fries	Slow cooker sweet potato curry served with one cup of cauliflower rice	Zucchini noodles with pesto and chicken	Orange chicken with roasted vegetables

In addition to this meal plan, here are a few helpful tips:

1. Make sure you have your own personal water bottle constantly so that you can stay hydrated.
2. Keep emergency snacks in your bag at all times so that you can eliminate any chance of getting too hungry during the day.

3. Do not skip your meals.
4. Limit your consumption of alcohol to 3 drinks per week or less.

FINAL WORDS...

Indeed, our diets have the power of affecting our health either positively or negatively; it all depends on our food choices. This book has explained that the earth is naturally endowed with foods for us to consume that will work with our bodies and provide us with essential nutrients we need to function properly and stay healthy. We introduced several superfoods and discussed their specific health benefits.

Surprisingly or not so surprisingly, each of these nutritional powerhouses has, to a certain extent, been scientifically proven to have specific medicinal advantages ranging from reducing the risk of various chronic diseases and boosting immunity to enhancing mental health and beauty. Perhaps, this might make you wonder why we often automatically resort to taking prescription medications before we consider making shifts in our diets to exploit the "powers" these superfoods have to offer us.

The reality is that we can improve our health by making better food choices and lifestyle adjustments, such as exercising regularly, decreasing alcohol consumption, or getting more sleep. By eating nutritious foods provided to us by the earth, rather than overly processed foods with little to no nutritious value, we can thwart off many diseases we commonly face. This does not have to be a difficult task. Use the tips provided in each chapter to start incorporating a superfood or two into each meal. Begin to cut back on the less healthy, overly processed food options.

You deserve to live a better and healthier life, so take that big step by making the best use of the tools readily available from this point onward! But just before you begin to walk the talk, kindly leave a review on Amazon if you enjoyed this book. We would also love to know about your growth as you progress with this new goal!

REFERENCES

Alleman, G.A. (2021). Ultimate Guide to Olive Oil. Retrieved from https://recipes.howstuffworks.com/how-olive-oil-works4.htm

Arnarson, A. (2019). Oranges 101: Nutrition Facts and Health Benefits. Retrieved from https://www.healthline.com/nutrition/foods/oranges

Austrasian Turkey Federation. (n.d.). Health benefits of eating turkey. Retrieved from https://www.turkeyfed.com.au/about-turkey/health-benefits/

Bray, M. (2019). Bell Pepper Benefits: How Healthy Are They? Retrieved from https://www.pepperscale.com/bell-pepper-benefits/

Brennan, D. (2020). Health Benefits of Mushrooms. Retrieved from https://www.webmd.com/diet/health-benefits-mushrooms#1

Butler, N. (2019). What to know about oranges. Retrieved from https://www.medicalnewstoday.com/articles/272782

Butler, N. (2017). Are Mushrooms Good for You? Retrieved from https://www.healthline.com/health/food-nutrition/are-mushrooms-good-for-you

Chilkov, N. (2011). Avocados: A Super Cancer Fighting Food. Retrieved from https://www.huffpost.com/entry/avocados-a-super-cancer-f_b_632985/amp

Choudhary, T. (2019). 22 Best Benefits Of Olive Oil For Skin, Hair, And Health. Retrieved from https://www.stylecraze.com/articles/amazing-benefits-of-olive-oil-that-you-never-knew/

De Thample, R. (2019). A Revolutionary Kitchen Ingredient: How To Cook With Kombucha. Retrieved from https://www.farmdrop.com/blog/how-to-cook-with-kombucha/

Dillon, K. (2021). Lime Water Vs Lemon Water Health Benefits: Which Is Better For You?. Retrieved from https://lajollamom.com/lemon-water-lime-water-health-benefits/

Dilmah Tea. (n.d.) NUTMEG. Retrieved from https://www.dilmahtea.com/herbal-infusion-tea/herbal-tea-benefits/nutmeg.html

Eckelkamp. S. (2021). 12 Surprising Health Benefits Of Olive Oil. Retrieved from https://www.aboutoliveoil.org/12-surprising-health-benefits-of-olive-oil

Girdwin, A. (2019). 6 Healthy Reasons Why Salmon Is a Staple of Practically Every Eating Plan Out There. Retrieved from https://www.wellandgood.com/health-benefits-of-salmon/

Hill, Ainsley. (2019). Lemons vs. Limes: What's the Difference? Retrieved from https://www.healthline.com/nutrition/lime-vs-lemon#similarities

Jennings, K. (2018). Top 9 Health Benefits of Eating Watermelon. Renieved from https://www.healthline.com/nutrition/watermelon-health-benefits

Julson, E. (2019). 6 Surprising Health Benefits of Sweet Potatoes. Retrieved from https://www.healthline.com/nutrition/sweet-potato-benefits

Kandora, A. (2019). What are the health benefits of lemons vs. limes? Retrieved from https://www.medicalnewstoday.com/articles/325228

Lam, P. (2020). What to know about anemia, Retrieved from https://www.medicalnewstoday.com/articles/158800#_noHeaderPrefixedContent

Lim, F. (2012). 6 EASY WAYS TO USE ONIONS IN YOUR MEALS. Retrieved from https://www.dishbydish.net/6-easy-ways-to-use-onions-in-your-meals/

Marengo, K. (2019). What is the nutritional value of mushrooms? Retrieved from https://www.medicalnewstoday.com/articles/278858

MasterClass. (2020). What Is Nutmeg? Learn How to Cook With Nutmeg. Retrieved from https://www.masterclass.com/articles/what-is-nutmeg-learn-how-to-cook-with-nutmeg#what-is-nutmeg

Meszaros, L. (2020). This popular fruit can protect against cancer and other dangerous diseases. Retrieved from https://www.mdlinx.com/article/this-popular-fruit-can protect-against-cancer-and-other-dangerous-diseases/6Pfjyzzaegb0uHGigN4Ihd

McCulloch, M. (2018). Are Sunflower Seeds Good for You? Nutrition, Benefits and More. Retrieved from https://www.healthline.com/nutrition/sunflower-seeds

Mikstas, C. (2019). 15 Healthy Ways to Use Lemons and Limes. Retrieved from https://www.webmd.com/food-recipes/ss/slideshow-lemons-and-limes

M & F Editor. (n.d.). 5 SURPRISING HEALTH BENEFITS OF TURKEY. Retrieved from https://www.muscleandfitness.com/nutrition/healthy-eating/5-surprising-health-benefits-turkey/

Rinkush. (n.d.) 13 Surprising Health Benefits of Chili Pepper You Absolutely Need to Know. Retrieved from https://www.conserve-energy-future.com/benefits-chili-pepper.php

Roy, A. (2019). 15 Health Benefits of Ginger: Skin, Hair and Recipes. Retrieved from https://www.medlife.com/blog/15-health-benefits-ginger-skin-hair-recipes/amp/

Robinson, K. (2019). What Are the Health Benefits of Avocado, and Can It Help You Lose Weight? Retrieved from https://www.everydayhealth.com/diet-nutrition/diet/avocados-health-benefits-nutrition-facts-weight-loss-info-more/

Saas, C. (2020). 7 Health Benefits of Oranges, According to a Nutritionist. Retrieved from https://www.health.com/food/health-benefits-oranges

Saas, C. (2020). 7 Health Benefits of Sweet Potatoes. Rerieved from https://www.health.com/nutrition/sweet-potato-health-benefits?amp=true

Sancha Tea Bar. (2020). Kombucha: Nutrition Facts, Health Benefits, and Dangers

of   This   Fermented   Tea.   Rerieved   from
https://senchateabar.com/blogs/blog/kombucha

Safebeat. (n.d.). 12 Health Benefits Of Salmon For The Heart, Brain, And Much
More.   Rerieved   from
https://safebeat.org/cardiac/heart health/12 health benefits of salmo
n for the heart brain and much more/

Salomon, S. H. (2019). What Is Cinnamon? A Comprehensive Guide to Using and
Reaping the Health Benefits of This Popular Ancient Spice. Rerieved from
https://www.everydayhealth.com/diet-nutrition/diet/cinnamon-
nutrition-benefits-types-recipes/

Shubrook, N. (2019). Top 6 health benefits of pumpkin seeds. Retrieved from
https://www.bbcgoodfood.com/howto/guide/health-benefits-pumpkin-
seeds/amp

Shubrook, N. (2018). The health benefits of broccoli. Retrieved from
https://www.bbcgoodfood.com/howto/guide/health-benefits-
broccoli/amp

ABOUT THE AUTHOR

I guess I'll say that I'm a gal who has gone against the grain as far
back in life as I can remember, but after realizing the nutritional
potency and healing power in foods, I've finally decided to start going
with the grains...yeah, and the vegetables and healthy fruits as well.

I wrote this book to take readers on a health journey with me. As a
pharmacist, I have seen just how the choices we make with our diets
can greatly impact our health and our lifestyle. Also, my mother, who
always seemed to be a vibrant, jubilant, healthy woman, was
diagnosed with and died of cancer at a relatively young age. This
event triggered my interest in food as a health resource and served as
a wake-up call that we humans can be very fragile.

In this book, I provide a dietary mechanism/roadmap for combatting
our fragility as humans to the greatest degree that we can dietarily. I
will discuss how certain foods can be our medicine. Please enjoy this
journey with me and make it your own!

www.ingramcontent.com/pod-product-compliance
Lightning Source LLC
Chambersburg PA
CBHW020258030426
42336CB00010B/822